AT YOUR BEST FOR BIRTH
AND LATER

AT YOUR BEST FOR BIRTH AND LATER

BY

EILEEN MONTGOMERY, M.C.S.P.

WITH A FOREWORD
BY

H. L. SHEPHERD, Ch.M., F.R.C.O.G.

Formerly Consultant Obstetrician and Gynæcologist, United Bristol Hospitals;
Lecturer in Obstetrics, University of Bristol

THIRD EDITION

BRISTOL: JOHN WRIGHT & SONS LTD.
1969

First published, December, 1959
Reprinted, July, 1962
Reprinted, May, 1963
Second Edition, July, 1964
Reprinted, October, 1966
Third Edition, June, 1969
Reprinted, June, 1974

ISBN 0 7236 0242 5

PRINTED IN GREAT BRITAIN BY JOHN WRIGHT & SONS LTD.
AT THE STONEBRIDGE PRESS, BRISTOL, BS4 5NU

PREFACE TO THE THIRD EDITION

IN the field of psychophysical preparation for childbirth, ideas which originated in Britain have been taken up and developed still further in other countries. Interest has spread to most parts of the world.

We are constantly progressing in the light of our own and other people's experience and research. Consequently, slight modifications and additions are necessary in this third edition.

The book was written primarily to assist prospective mothers—who should carry out the advice with the approval of their doctor or nurse/midwife—but it drew appreciative comments from qualified as well as lay readers.

In recent years the Royal College of Midwives and other professional bodies responsible for the care and instruction of mothers have arranged postgraduate courses and invited me to pass on the techniques described in this book from the teacher's point of view.

If the attendants in labour understand what the mother is trying to do—even if they themselves have not trained her beforehand—the benefits will be reinforced. It gives young parents great confidence to know that positive support and, if necessary, a little prompting will be given.

We hope the additions will be helpful to *all* readers.

E. M.

Bristol, 1969

ACKNOWLEDGEMENTS

My interest in training for childbirth was kindled by Miss Minnie Randall, O.B.E., S.R.N., S.C.M., F.C.S.P. (Hon.). Later it was increased while producing my own family and by the teaching of the late Mrs. Helen Heardman, F.C.S.P. (Hon.). Since then, it has been sustained constantly by watching and listening to many doctors and midwives with a wealth of experience and a variety of points of view. To them all I am indebted.

Numerous mothers, both prepared and unprepared for labour, have by their comments, personal observations, and behaviour taught me a great deal and I am grateful to them.

It has been a privilege to work in a medical and midwifery teaching hospital where there is such excellent co-operation and unity of purpose among the members of the staff. All have in some measure been responsible for this harmony, but Miss N. B. Deane, C.B.E., Past President of the Royal College of Midwives and Matron of Bristol Maternity Hospital, has set the keynote.

I wish to express my thanks especially to Mr. H. L. Shepherd, F.R.C.O.G., formerly Consultant Obstetrician and Gynæcologist to the United Bristol Hospitals, for his advice and guidance and for writing a foreword to this book.

My appreciation is also due to Mrs. Jean Gifford, M.C.S.P., and Miss Barbara Shotton, M.C.S.P., for reading the manuscript and suggesting some rearrangement of the text; to Mrs. Geraldine Buffery for her black silhouette figure drawings, and to the publishers, John Wright & Sons Ltd., for their interest and efficiency in the handling and reproduction of the subject matter.

CONTENTS

NOTES

FOREWORD TO THE FIRST EDITION

FOR many years Mrs. Montgomery has been a most valued member of the Staff of the Bristol Maternity Hospital.

During this time I have learned to appreciate the great benefits which her work has given to thousands of patients, both to their mental and physical comfort and to their safety at the time of childbirth. How much these benefits have been due to the physical methods and the physiological education which patients learn at her Relaxation Classes, and how much to the confidence which she herself inspires, I have always found it hard to decide, but only a mistress of her subject could have gained the success she has.

I was, therefore, pleased when she told me that she had decided to write *At Your Best for Birth*. It is always a difficult task to reduce to print a subject which is essentially a personal matter between Instructor and Patient, but she has succeeded and I feel sure that this small book will not only be of value and interest to Expectant Mothers but also to Midwives and Members of the Medical Profession.

H. L. SHEPHERD, F.R.C.O.G.

Bristol Maternity Hospital,
  October, 1959.

AT YOUR BEST FOR BIRTH
AND LATER

I. INTRODUCTION

The Evolution of the Theme.—
Many doctors and midwives have found that education with certain physical exercises and training in relaxation before childbirth is an investment which pays dividends when the baby is born and later on —but not all.

Some remark: "We have tried it and it does not seem to us to make much difference" or words to that effect. But have they in mind the same type of preparation ? Even the word 'relaxation' can mean either 'diminution of tension' or 'diversion', and 'training in relaxation' can also represent different things to different people.

In some places isolated instructors, having little or no contact with the person who will conduct the delivery of the baby, concentrate on the physical training and relaxation of the expectant mother—and this is probably of little value alone—whereas in others the aim is not only to obtain her physical but mental and emotional relaxation as well. Where this is achieved 'teaching relaxation' is considered to be more than worth while both by the mothers and those who come into contact with them.

In the 1930's, Fairbairn included prenatal instruction as part of the scope of his unit at St. Thomas's Hospital, London. He was of the opinion that more should be done on the preventive side and he called this 'constructive physiology'. He looked upon prenatal relaxation and exercise in the same light as the drill of a soldier. "They are a discipline in the power of control under stress which, if once attained, will give that confidence that is half the battle."

Kathleen Vaughan, whose influence was felt in the same unit, worked for many years as an obstetrician in Kashmir. She had found that those women who led an active life in the open air had their babies easily, whereas those who lived in purdah with its strict rules on seclusion had very little exercise or sunlight and they delivered their babies with difficulty.

She maintained that in the West, as in the East, the more confined and artificial the way of life, the greater the complications of child-bearing, and she initiated exercise classes in London with the aim of helping town-bred, civilized women to have their babies naturally and easily. To do this she found that three things are necessary: (1) A well-developed and normally shaped pelvis; (2) Flexible joints in the pelvis; and (3) An unconstrained attitude for delivery.

Maybe our little girls and adolescents should learn the type of pelvic movement which she advocated, for once maturity is reached the shape of the pelvis cannot be altered by exercise.

At about the same time Dick Read, another British pioneer, popularized the theory that fear leads to tension, which in turn causes pain in childbirth. His first principle therefore of obtaining what he called 'a natural birth' was that all fear and tension should be eradicated and confidence built up.

Some of those influenced by his teaching have called the techniques involved 'natural childbirth training' and others, while approving of most of his methods, do not quite accept the implications in this label, since natural birth often occurs spontaneously in untrained women and a few of those who *have* been trained need medical assistance in labour.

During the last few years a new word 'psychoprophylaxis' has appeared in our vocabulary. It was coined by Nicolaiev in 1949 to classify a system which, it is claimed, originated in Russia. In 1951, with two colleagues, Velvovsky and Platonov, he explained and demonstrated the method at a medical conference in Leningrad. It spread quickly across Europe and Asia and though the *theory* differs from the earlier methods of prenatal preparation which were developed in Great Britain, the practical applications are very similar.

Briefly there are two elements involved in psychoprophylaxis. The first is based on Pavlov's theory of conditioned reflexes. Probably his best-known experiment was in conditioning dogs. Every time the dogs were fed, a bell was rung, until eventually he had only to ring the bell without producing the food and the dogs began to dribble. They now associated food with a signal—the sound of a bell.

So the Russians maintain that we have been conditioned over a very long period (by hearsay, books, films, etc.) to associate pain with childbirth. That it is not, in fact, an inborn attribute of women and that by de-conditioning these pernicious associations and re-conditioning with beneficial ones (education about the working and pattern of normal childbirth, building up of confidence, and sustained support) pain rarely becomes a problem.

Their second element is based on a focus of activity to raise the pain threshold. If you have ever been in a crowded railway train you will be aware that your brain is incapable of appreciating both the contents of a book *and* the conversation of the other passengers. If you are sufficiently engrossed in your book the talk does not register.

Football, Rugby, and Hockey players, in the intensity of the game, do not notice the minor injuries to which they are subjected and women in labour, if given a programme of physical and mental activity, which demands a focus for their concentration, can 'block' the painful stimuli from reaching that part of the brain where they become conscious.

Many practitioners are finding in the light of experience that both the British and Continental types of combined physical and mental training can produce similarly satisfactory results; but the intensity of the instruction given must be sufficient to break down faulty associations with childbearing—whether we call them fears or conditioned reflexes—and build up sound ones.

Neither method should be regarded as an alternative to analgesics (pain relievers) and medication during labour, but the need for them is lessened. Heavy sedation will, of course, dull the power to concentrate on a focus of activity, but the lighter sedatives can soothe a patient who remains alert and active should the necessity arise.

Since patterns of living and behaviour, individual temperaments, and midwifery techniques vary somewhat from country to country and place to place, so perhaps no method will be wholly acceptable to everybody, everywhere. The course outlined here does not adhere rigidly to any particular authority. It has evolved logically and is adaptable to its environment.

A ship's captain has learnt his seamanship; passengers and crew have confidence in his ability, yet, when nearing port, he hands over the control of navigation to a pilot more familiar with the channels, currents, tides, and other natural forces. So the woman who is instructed along the following lines and who practises regularly the exercises set to improve her 'know-how' will be able to ride the waves of labour more skilfully, yet adapt herself where necessary to the directions of her pilot/attendant according to her special needs.

Ideally, doctor, midwife, physiotherapist, and mother work together as a team to maintain and strengthen, as far as possible, the normal design for childbearing. Often, under different circumstances, there may be only two members of the team, midwife and mother working together with complete understanding. In this way the conditions—tangible and intangible—are at the best possible.

The Fundamentals.—

Most men and women have experienced that feeling of acute uneasiness immediately before going to a new school, entering for an examination, or awaiting an important interview. Facing an unknown ordeal makes us anxious, tense, and braced up. Our internal organs also are affected. The rhythm of the heart-beat quickens, breathing becomes shallow and irregular, and appetite is lost. We talk of having 'butterflies in the tummy' and there may be an irritating effect on the bladder.

An unprepared woman coming into labour for the first time may react in a similar manner. She does not know what to expect or what will be expected of her. The bladder lies immediately in front of the uterus (the muscular organ where the baby grows and which, when the time is ready, will contract to propel him into the outside world) and the same nerves supply the two organs. We can appreciate, then, that if emotional tension has upset the muscular control of the bladder, it can also under similar circumstances upset the muscular control of the uterus.

Confidence, with consequent easing of tension and settling down of internal rhythm, comes with foreknowledge of how to deal with any situation that might arise. When a woman knows how to help herself and co-operate as requested—how to relax or exert her muscles in the right way and at the right time—the whole process of pregnancy, birth, and restoration to full activity is usually smoother and much more satisfactory to the mother and to everybody concerned.

So, since emotional tension leads to physical tension, it is of prime importance to learn, in addition to control of the body and relaxation, enough about the physiology of labour to eliminate the anxiety and uncertainty from the mind. Beforehand, the prospective mother should be made aware of what sensory and visible milestones she may encounter at the beginning and throughout the three stages of labour, and of the ministrations that are likely to be carried out as a routine by the midwifery and medical attendants.

The Right Approach to Childbirth.—

The expectant mother should consult her doctor or midwife early in pregnancy. The sooner the plans and arrangements for the confinement are made, whether at home or away, the better.

She should be ready to have a check-up from time to time during pregnancy and, unless her husband is away from home, to talk over with him any discussion that has taken place, so that both may understand the reasons for and stand by any advice given.

At successive meetings between patient and doctor or midwife, each understands the other better, so that when labour is in progress, the patient is at ease and confident in their skill and the doctor or midwife has a more confident approach to the patient.

In addition, the woman who has had pre-natal instruction and has practised controlled breathing and relaxation has more confidence in herself. She knows how to help and how to co-operate in the conduct of her labour, whether quick or slow, to the best of her own ability. This is a great advantage.

II. BASIC PHYSIOLOGY

To grasp what happens during pregnancy and labour we must know, first, a little about the uterus and birth-canal, and, secondly, about the pelvis, the bone structure in the lower part of the trunk.

The *Uterus* (*Fig.* 1 A) is shaped like an upturned flagon, with its upper part tilted forwards towards the abdominal wall, and its bottle-neck (the cervix) opening into the *Vagina*, the lower part of the birth-canal through which the baby will emerge. Throughout pregnancy there is a mucus plug in the *Cervix* which seals it up like a stopper.

Until he is born, the *Foetus*—the term for the unborn baby—does not breathe, eat, or excrete, yet he needs oxygen and food while he is developing. These two essentials are carried to him through the *Placenta*, which grows like roots into the thickened walls of the uterus. Nutrient substances are taken from the mother's blood in much the same way as the root of a water plant derives sustenance. These are carried along the *Cord* by a blood-vessel to circulate around the baby's body. His waste and carbon dioxide are collected in two other vessels and flow back along the cord via his navel, and so back to the placenta and into the mother's blood-stream, to be dealt with by her kidneys and lungs.

The foetus is suspended in watery fluid inside filmy-thin but very strong membranes. This liquor keeps the temperature even, and acts as a shock absorber. In the event of a fall, though the mother may be shaken, baby is protected.

Early in pregnancy, the walls of the uterus thicken and develop more and more muscle-tissue. Muscle, anywhere in the body, is like living elastic. As it contracts, it becomes shorter and thicker, and as it relaxes, it gets longer and thinner. There are circular muscle-fibres in the lower segment of the uterus—like the draw-thread of a sponge bag—which keep it closed until the baby is ready to be born. There are also longitudinal muscle-fibres stretched from the *Fundus*—the extreme upper part of the uterus—over the upper segment and down the opposite side towards the cervix. For comparison, think of the geographical lines of longitude and latitude on the globe. The difference is that whereas on the world they are spaced at regular intervals between the north and south poles, in the uterus the longitudinal muscle-fibres are much more abundant and closer together in the upper segment, and the circular fibres are much closer together in the lower segment.

In labour, as each strand of longitudinal muscle contracts, it gathers up the smooth tissue of the uterine walls and draws the lower segment upwards over the baby's head, while the circular fibres relax and allow the cervix to be opened (*Fig.* 1 B). If there is excessive emotional tension, the circular fibres may be less responsive and the consequent resistance can prolong labour and cause unnecessary discomfort. Unfortunately, if a patient is already scared and the next contraction proves even more uncomfortable, her emotional tension is not likely to ease! A vicious circle is established which may prove difficult to break.

It is this *unnecessary* resistance, and the pain which sometimes results, that can be reduced during the first stage of labour. Emotional relaxation can be maintained in early labour by being contentedly occupied, and in the later first stage by easy rhythmical breathing and physical relaxation, so that birth is accomplished with the maximum of ease and the minimum of pain and fatigue.

The greatest amount of power is exerted at the fundus of the uterus. Contraction in this area squeezes the contents down towards the lower

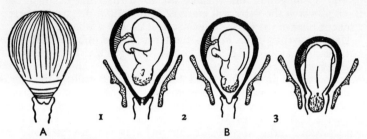

Fig. 1.—Diagram of the uterus. A, The uterus, showing longitudinal and circular muscle-fibres. B, Dilatation of the cervix and spiral descent of baby through the pelvis. 1, At onset of first stage: mucus plug in cervix; membranes intact; baby's head in brim of pelvis. 2, First stage: cervix about half dilated; membranes bulging; baby's head midway down in pelvis. 3, During second stage: cervix fully dilated; membranes ruptured, baby's head descending lower part of birth-canal and passing through outlet of pelvis.

segment, just as by squeezing the extreme end of a tube of tooth-paste the contents are pushed towards the nozzle.

Uterine muscle, unlike other muscle, has the power of retraction, i.e., that having shortened on contraction, the fibres do not lengthen again on coming to rest, and progressive shortening takes place. With much the same effect, having pressed some tooth-paste on to the brush each time we use it, we roll the empty portion of the tube towards the bulk and in this way we keep an even pressure exerted in the direction of the outlet.

The *Vagina* tilts at right angles to the uterus and, because of the corrugated nature of its walls, is capable of prodigious stretching during the second stage of labour, when the baby descends it in a forward and downward direction.

The *Pelvis (Fig.* 2) has been compared to a bony basin. This is kept balanced at its correct tilt by the muscles of the abdominal wall, which pull the front of the basin upward, and the muscles of the seat, which pull the back of the basin downward. There are two joints at the back of the pelvis where the spine meets the 'basin' (the sacro-iliac joints). Here some movement takes place with certain changes of position throughout life. There is one joint in front (the pubic symphysis) which moves only during pregnancy and childbearing.

A hormone (chemical), called *Relaxin*, is liberated into the blood-stream during pregnancy and this causes the ligaments, which beforehand bound these joints together tightly, to become more relaxed. The pelvis is thus enabled to give slightly in front at the pubic joint, and in

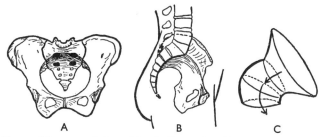

Fig. 2.—Diagrams of the pelvis. A, Front view; B, Side view, section; C, Comparison to a flue.

the back at the two sacro-iliac joints. Forward and backward swivel action is thus permitted, which, though it reduces the stability of the joints, increases the width of the birth-canal.

Immediately after birth this hormone disappears from the blood and the ligaments and joints gradually return to normal.

Neuromuscular Control.—

Exercise is a means by which muscular control and tone are developed. If the tone is good, then, like the best elastic, muscle will stretch sufficiently, maintain support, and spring back to its original position. If the tone is poor, then it is similar to the cheap sort of elastic which stretches too much, fails to support properly, and loses its power of recoil.

Athletes talk of being 'fit'. They mean that their bodies are at the peak of physical perfection. In such condition, there is no need for conscious control of muscle to maintain correct posture or to execute their particular form of physical prowess. Their method becomes automatic. But to have reached such a state of fitness, there must have been a period of training, when not once, but many times a particular posture or movement was consciously studied, with the senses keyed to assess either an increase or a reduction of fatigue or strain.

Performance of a few exercises once or twice a day cannot produce this tone if, during the rest of the day, we are standing, walking, and sitting around with faulty posture. The mind becomes attuned to the slouch or the over-braced carriage and we are then no longer aware of our faults, though we *are* aware of the aches resulting from our fatigue.

We can, however, attune our minds to the correct use of the body in everyday life. By consciously appreciating how it feels to us when we stand, walk, sit, or perform certain movements the *right* way, we develop what is known as the postural reflex. We then automatically correct ourselves.

Fatigue and how to reduce it.—When a fuel is burnt, it leaves some form of ash or residue. In doing so, it has created energy or heat. When a muscle works it also uses fuel from the blood-stream (oxygen and nutritional substances), and produces waste and carbon dioxide.

During muscle contraction, the blood-vessels are squeezed and the blood-supply is diminished. Contraction is usually followed by relaxation and a fresh blood-supply then rushes through the now dilated blood-vessels, to carry away the waste products. When a muscle is called upon to work without rest, the waste collects sufficiently to irritate the nerve-endings in the locality. This causes an ache.

On holiday, we sometimes require the calf muscles of our legs to work much harder than usual. We set out to walk up a steep hill or climb a cliff path. After a while, the calves ache—waste products have collected in that area, there is pressure on nerve-endings with consequent fatigue—and we want to rest. While we sit down by the wayside, the ache gradually subsides, the waste is carried away by the blood-stream, replaced by freshly oxygenated blood, and within a short time we are able to continue up the incline, without discomfort.

It will be obvious, then, that by performing our daily routine in positions which reduce muscle work to a minimum we shall also reduce fatigue. This applies equally to men and women in all walks of life.

There is an upper control in the brain which regulates the rate of breathing, so that the oxygen intake is at the correct rate for the demands of the body. Consequently, when we work our muscles hard we automatically breathe more deeply and more quickly, since they are using up more oxygen.

In pregnancy and labour the mother's lungs have to provide enough oxygen for the baby's needs in addition to her own. Her blood collects the baby's waste products, too, so that her kidneys are called upon to do more work than before. The mother's body must deal with these extra demands for her baby. The answer, then, is to learn to discipline oneself to cut out unnecessary fatigue.

This does not mean becoming completely idle and cutting out all forms of physical effort. Certain breathing exercises and smooth rhythmic movements are extremely beneficial, but they should be alternated with periods of complete rest.

III. THE PREPARATION

1.—POSTURE, POISE, AND COMFORT IN DAILY LIVING—BEFORE AND AFTER BIRTH

By standing, working, and walking correctly, and also getting our proper quota of rest, we minimize the stresses and strains on our bodies and we look more graceful (*Fig.* 3 B). As pregnancy progresses and the weight of the baby increases, there may be a tendency to stand with a hollow back and the pelvic basin tipping forward (*Fig.* 3 A). This

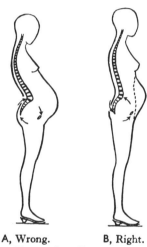

A, Wrong.   B, Right.
Fig. 3.—Standing posture.

tendency must be resisted! If we allow ourselves to stand in this way the weight of the baby will tip the pelvis forward off balance (like a see-saw), and even greater strain will be thrown on the lower abdominal wall and the joints between the lower spine and the pelvis. The hollow-backed standing position is the commonest cause of backache in pregnancy, which, if the habit sticks, may persist for years.

The more the weight of the baby is thrown forward, the greater the strain on the abdominal muscles. Yet, these should be used as Nature intended, to hold the front of the pelvis up, while the buttocks keep the back of it down. Unfortunately, the more stretched the abdominal muscles get, the more they lose their ability to do this job efficiently. The weight of the baby may then fall forward out of the basin into soft tissues instead of being carried mainly on bone.

Such an attitude may also lead to troublesome feet. The thigh bones are rotated inwards, and the body-weight is transmitted to the inner instead of towards the outer borders of the feet. Already having to carry more weight than usual, they are thus subjected to an even greater strain, and fallen arches can result.

Stand this way (and occasionally check yourself in a mirror):—

1. Feet slightly apart and facing forward, with weight towards the outer borders, midway between the heels and the balls of the feet.
2. Knees straight but not braced back hard, knee-caps facing forward.
3. Front of pelvis up. (Seat muscles braced and lower abdominal wall lifted, then partially relaxed, so that the balance is maintained.)
4. Rib cage lifted upwards and outwards.
5. Shoulders relaxed.
6. Head and neck upright, as if being pulled upward like a puppet on a string, attached to the top of the head.

Common Faults in Walking.—

The head is rather like a heavy football being balanced on a pole. When it is allowed to drop forward, the muscles at the back of the neck have to work constantly to prevent it going even further forward, and this causes an ache. Yet, many people walk in this way, looking at the ground a few feet in front of them (*Fig.* 4 A).

The forward dropping head leads to Fault No. 2: the sternum (breast-bone) and ribs become depressed and the shoulders are rounded. Now the normal curves of the spine will be accentuated and the abdomen and pelvis will tend to drop forward (Fault No. 3). In such a position the swing in walking must be from the knees instead of the hips (Fault No. 4) and the thighs are rotated inwards, throwing the weight too much on the inner borders of the feet, with the toes turned outward (Fault No. 5). How one fault leads to another! A vicious spiral indeed!

How do you walk? Are any of these faults your faults? Let us make sure by taking everything in turn:—

1. Start off in the correct standing position as in *Fig.* 3 B. The head should be upright, the neck straight so that its muscles can easily maintain the heavy skull at its correct alinement, mostly by balance. Sense that the weight of the body is correctly placed on the feet and that the knee-caps are forward.
2. Abdomen should be held up with seat tucked down and under sufficiently to balance the pelvis.
3. The rib cage and chest should be well up and wide but shoulders relaxed (not braced back like a guardsman). Now breathing is easy and uninhibited.
4. Swing forward from the hips and place the feet down straight. The weight of the body should be transmitted first to the heels, then to the outer borders, from there to the balls of the feet. Lastly, push off with the big toes.

The head need not be allowed to drop again in order to look at the feet. In walking correctly, the eyes can be dropped occasionally, while keeping the head erect (*Fig.* 4 B).

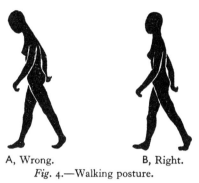

A, Wrong.   B, Right.
Fig. 4.—Walking posture.

Consider your posture and gait
Whenever you're having to wait.

How do you sit? On the edge of the chair with only the upper part of the thighs supported and a gap between the lower spine and the back of the chair?
Again, one fault will lead to another. Abdomen sags, breast bone and ribs are depressed. There will be back strain and a greater chance of

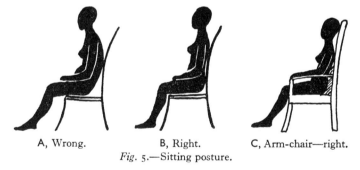

A, Wrong.   B, Right.   C, Arm-chair—right.
Fig. 5.—Sitting posture.

suffering from indigestion, since all the contents of the abdomen are compressed unnecessarily (*Fig.* 5 A).
Feel the difference when sitting correctly. Sit well back on the chair so that the whole length of the thighs is supported—buttocks right back against the chair-back or cushion (*Fig.* 5 B).
In an arm-chair the tendency to sit badly is even greater. Only recently have furniture manufacturers realized that men and women need different fittings! How many women at the end of a day's work, when rest is required, sit drooping back in an arm-chair with the lower

back unsupported, or, because that is uncomfortable, perch sideways, resting one side of their spine against the arm of the chair, with shoulders hunched forward and neck tensed, knitting, sewing, or watching television.

By placing a cushion behind the back in such a way as to reduce the distance from front to back, then sitting down with seat well back, we gain the support that we need to relax properly (*Fig.* 5 C).

How do you do the washing-up, the cake- and pastry-making, and the cooking? Do you stand with the feet side by side and the head and shoulders bent forward, so that there is continuous back strain in one locality (*Fig.* 6 A)?

Better to stand with one foot slightly in front of the other so that you sway slightly backwards and forwards. Make sure that your working surfaces are at the correct height for your own comfort: about 20 in. down from the shoulders (approximately wrist-level) is the correct height for most people (*Fig.* 6 B).

If your sink has a built-in cupboard underneath it, so that you cannot put one foot forward when facing it, turn slightly towards the draining board. If it is too low and cannot be raised, bend slightly from the knees or use a duck-board underneath the washing-up bowl.

How do you use a vacuum cleaner, carpet-sweeper, broom, or mop? If right-handed, place the left foot well in front of the right and use the body to sway from the hips, backwards and forwards (right foot forward if left-handed, *Fig.* 6 C). The back foot should be straight, so that it can be used to give forward thrust. The diagonal pull across the body from the left to right with a firm base makes movement easier and gives additional power, e.g., tennis, badminton, and squash players place the left foot forward when serving or striking with the right hand.

When pushing furniture, stand close up to it with one foot well in front of the other and back foot straight. Bend slightly from the knees and hips, keeping the trunk upright, and push forward with both hands, using your body-weight and thrust from back foot.

Similarly when pulling, the body-weight should be used, with knees relaxed and arms straight.

Tight skirts should not be worn for housework or you will find it impossible to carry out these suggestions.

How do you bend down to pick things up, look in the oven, tuck in the bedclothes, lift up the toddler? Are your legs straight, thus placing all the effort on the spinal muscles, often the cause of the all-too-common slipped disk (*Fig.* 6 D)? Or do you bend from the knees and hips as the champion weight lifters do, putting the main effort on the thigh muscles by straightening the knees and pushing the feet firmly against the floor (*Fig.* 6 E, F, and G)?

Keep bulky objects like washing baskets or grocery delivery boxes as near to the body as possible, and use the knee as a lever on which to rest one corner of the object and help to raise it. Never try to lift a dustbin when it is full.

While you are pregnant, and until you have fully recovered the strength of your abdominal and pelvic muscles afterwards, it is unwise to lift *heavy* weights anyway, but for the tasks about the house that most women expect to continue doing, remember that footwork is important. Sporting experts know that with their feet correctly placed, giving a

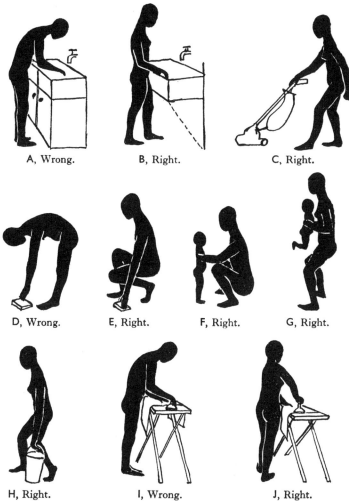

A, Wrong.   B, Right.   C, Right.

D, Wrong.   E, Right.   F, Right.   G, Right.

H, Right.   I, Wrong.   J, Right.

Fig. 6.—How to go about the housework : A, B, Washing-up ; C, Vacuum cleaning ; D, E, Lifting light object ; F, G, Picking up child ; H, Lifting heavy object at side ; I, J, Ironing.

firm base, they have even greater strength, with freedom of movement. So have you!

When lifting fairly heavy objects with a handle, e.g., buckets, coal scuttles, watering cans, etc., place the left foot forward and have the object to be lifted on the right side midway between the left and the right foot (*Fig.* 6 H). Bend the knees, keeping the spine straight, grasp the handle with the right hand, push the feet against the floor and walk forward with head up and neck straight. (If lifting with the left hand, have the object on your left side and place the right foot forward.)

When you do the ironing or polish the furniture, do not stand as in *Fig.* 6 I, but keep one foot in front or diagonally and use the opposite arm, twisting the trunk or swaying back and forth, using the body-weight (*Fig.* 6 J). In this way the chores actually become beneficial.

Notes on Comfort in Pregnancy.—

SHOES.—Wear comfortable shoes. It really depends on the height of the instep and the elasticity of the tendon at the back of the heel whether low or medium-high heels are preferable. Some women are made positively miserable by wearing flat shoes if they have not done so for years. Two things are certain: (1) Very high or narrow heels make it impossible to stand or walk correctly. (2) No shoes, even low shoes, should ever be sloppy at the instep. Choose an easy fit for toes and front arch and a firm fit at the instep.

EXTRA SUPPORTS.—A woman who is able to maintain sound posture will not need any extra support in the way of a maternity corset. Keeping stockings up may be a problem, but garters should never be worn. They compress the veins of the legs, causing congestion of blood and adding to fatigue. Avoid also the suspender belt which pulls downward from the waist and the tight girdle which compresses.

If at any time it is found to be impossible to hold the pelvis up in front, or if, when nobody is looking, there is a desire to place the hands underneath the 'bump' to take the weight, a maternity support should be worn. It should lift the lower abdomen, correct the pelvic tilt, and reduce the back strain without constricting.

A good brassière is an investment. During pregnancy the breasts develop extra cells which secrete a substance called 'colostrum'. Later on, after the baby is born, these cells will be ready to produce milk. The growth of tissue, sometimes rapid, will increase the weight and size of the breasts. In the erect posture, gravity pulls downward on the breasts. If they are heavy and are allowed to sag, overstretching of the supportive tissues may result. Imagine the damage which may be done to the line of the figure by walking (or using a vacuum cleaner) with an inadequate brassière or none at all!

Be conscious always that the weight of the bosom is suspended as in a sling from the shoulders, even when bending sideways. Many women are advised to wear a brassière in bed and are much more comfortable when doing so. If we prevent sagging, we shall help to preserve the rounded contour and keep, and perhaps improve, the figure.

Choose a garment with a firm diaphragm band underneath the cups, and with adequate shoulder straps. Narrow shoulder straps sometimes cause furrows on the flesh over the shoulders. The garment which fits one woman may not be right for another. Styles and figures vary, and it is essential to try on before purchasing.

The cups should give a good separation of the breasts without squeezing outward or inward and be of the right width and depth to give adequate support.

N.B.—Remember the tip about putting your brassière on and fastening up while bending the trunk forward, so that the breasts fall forward and not downwards into the cups.

Towards the end of pregnancy, colostrum sometimes leaks slightly. If this happens, do not be persuaded to buy a brassière with rubber or plastic shields. The non-porous material prevents the skin from 'breathing'; warmth from the body condenses on the inside and this can cause irritation or soreness. To give protection if necessary, wear small squares of turkish towelling, kept scrupulously clean, or of 'gamgee' tissue (thin cotton-wool, sandwiched between two layers of gauze), inside the brassière.

CARE OF THE SKIN.—Skins vary greatly in their ability to stretch without damage. Some contain more elastic tissue, and their owners are the lucky ones who can produce twins and keep a smooth yet firmly springy abdomen.

Though there is an element of luck in the type of skin we are born with, there is a method of helping the skin to stretch better, and of reducing the chances of getting striæ gravidarum—those permanent silvery wrinkles, reddish during pregnancy, which some women notice too late!

From about 4–5 months in pregnancy, with the first sign of a change in contour, start this treatment two or three times a week. After hot (not too hot) baths, when the skin has been dried, pour a *small* amount of almond or olive oil into the palms of hands and work well into the skin over the abdomen, hips, buttocks, and upper thighs.

The massage technique is important: Pick up a 'wave' of skin between the index finger and the thumb of both hands and by sliding over the oily surface, roll it so that the 'wave' moves downwards, upwards, and sideways, over all the parts mentioned. This preparation will also prevent irritation of the abdominal wall due to the stretching which some women find annoying towards the end of pregnancy.

A little oil will work right in. It is not beneficial to leave oneself in a soggy mess through using a larger quantity. When you have finished, there will be a slight oiliness left on the hands. Use it with a gentle upward stroke on the under surface of the breasts. Never allow downward pressure to be used here, for fear of stretching the delicate supports and the pectoral muscles which help to anchor the breasts to the shoulders.

Circulatory Pressure Points.—

There are veins on the inside of the thighs which carry blood from the feet and legs back towards the heart. They join up to form one large vessel in the pelvis, just below the place where the baby is carried. In the standing position, unfortunately, gravity pulls the weight of the baby downwards and the pressure may fall continuously on the same area of this large vein. There will then be a traffic block; blood containing waste will be held up in the pelvis and consequently there will be back pressure right down the veins of the legs to the feet.

This is one of the aggravating causes of varicose veins and hæmorrhoids (piles), and if they are in the family—there is a certain amount of hereditary predisposition—they are more likely to occur in pregnancy than at any other time of life.

By moving, we vary the pressure points, but standing for long periods is detrimental.

Cramp in the legs may also be due to diminished blood-supply to the muscles (usually the calf muscles).

Relief.—Prevention is better than cure. Therefore do your utmost to maintain a good blood-supply to the legs by changing the position of the body. Walking is an excellent form of exercise.

If cramp does occur, it is relieved by stretching the muscle, which is in a state of involuntary contraction. If the calf muscle is affected, then, keeping the knee absolutely straight, grasp the foot and bend it upwards as hard as possible. To improve the circulation to the whole leg bend

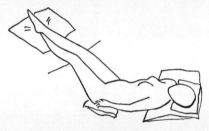

Fig. 7.—Reclining with the feet higher than the pelvis.

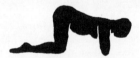

Fig. 8.—Knee–forearm prone kneeling (to relieve backache and circulatory congestion).

and stretch the toes and ankles and roll the foot round and round in circles. Do this lying down, before settling down for the night.

People who have developed varicose veins usually say that *before* the veins became swollen, their legs felt very tired and heavy, sometimes almost numb. This, I feel sure, is Nature's warning. It should be a signal to stand as little as possible and to rest in a favourable position more frequently.

Doctors usually advise lying down and putting the feet up higher than the pelvis (*Fig.* 7) or sleeping with the foot of the bed slightly raised so that the return of blood is assisted towards the heart by the incline. This is not always possible, if we are just in the middle of preparing a meal and the legs begin to feel heavy; but there is another position which will also relieve pressure on pelvic veins. Kneel down on all fours with hands directly under shoulders and knees directly under hips, then bend elbows and place forearms on the floor where the hands were previously (*Fig.* 8).

The weight of the baby in this position will be slipping up the trunk towards the shoulders and within a couple of minutes there will be a completely fresh blood-supply in the legs.

On getting up again, the legs will feel lighter and you will be able to continue with renewed energy.

Nerve Pressure Points.—

Towards the end of pregnancy, an ache sometimes occurs in the back, hips, or thighs, particularly when the standing position is maintained for longish periods. This may be due to pressure of the baby on small nerves on the inside of the vertebrae and pelvis.

Relief.—By kneeling on all fours, the weight of the baby will be tipped off those little nerves and his weight will be transmitted towards the upper front of the abdominal wall. Most backaches in pregnancy will be relieved simply by adopting this prone kneeling position for a short time.

Diaphragm Pressure.—

At between 6 and 8 months, when the baby is high in the abdomen, the diaphragm is compressed against the bases of the lungs. This occasionally causes a temporary pressure-pain, like cramp or 'stitch', under the ribs.

Relief.—Lift the rib cage by raising the arms sideways and upwards above the head. Stretch the spine and 'grow taller'.

Eight-point Plan for Comfort and Ease.—

1. Stand still as little as possible. Use the following positions for working and gardening wherever convenient:—
    a. Sitting on a chair with thighs and lower back fully supported or sitting on a stool with feet supported.
    b. Kneeling on all fours.
    c. Kneeling and sitting back on heels with thighs apart.
    d. Kneeling on one knee.
    e. Squatting (*see Fig.* 17, p. 46).
2. Wear suitable clothing and footwear.
3. Watch your posture with a critical eye and think about the position of the feet before starting any job.
4. Take your routine easily—dashing about only frays tempers and makes us more tired and less effective—and alternate hard work with more restful jobs.
5. Relax completely with the feet up to split the day and refresh for the evening.
6. Get plenty of fresh air and sunshine, but be wise and start sun-bathing in small doses in the summer.
7. Be moderate in all things. Eat a balanced diet. Your doctor or midwife will advise you on this.
8. Enjoy life.

2.—RELAXATION AND BREATHING CONTROL

Certain emotional reactions change the rate of respiration. Have you not become aware of yourself (or somebody else) breathing quickly when frightened, excited, or in a temper?

By keeping our breathing regular and easy, we help to steady our emotions and to relax mentally.

It is not beneficial to overbreathe—bearing in mind that delicate upper control previously mentioned which looks after the respiratory rate—in fact by so doing we can cause giddiness.

Basic Breathing Exercise.—

Position.—Sitting down, thighs and spine fully supported as in *Fig.* 5 B or C (p. 21). Place the hands on the front of the abdominal wall just above the waist and let the elbows rest on the arms of the chair or down to the side.

Movement.—Breathe in through the nose calmly—feel the air going low down into the lungs, expanding the abdominal wall underneath the hands.

When ready to breathe out, just let go and sigh through the nose or blow gently, making the sort of noise which expresses sheer bliss or relief. When another breath is required, breathe in again—low down, easily—without holding it, and concentrate on letting chest and shoulders go completely slack on breathing out (making a similar noise). Allow the lungs to deflate as much as they want to and they will inflate again, quite naturally, without your conscious thought!

Within a short time, each individual will have found her own natural rhythm. Notice the calming and soothing effect that it has.

Relaxation.—

Some people can relax all their muscles completely; some find it extremely difficult: others *think* they are relaxed when, in fact, there is still evident tension in certain muscles.

Those in the first group need no instruction; those in the second and third can be trained to relax, if they can learn to recognize the slight but quite definite sensations which are always present when muscle is tensed or contracted.

These sensations in the muscles and tendons themselves can be felt, not only when a part of the body is moved obviously but also when muscles are merely braced, without apparent movement. When muscles contract, they behave like living elastic, so there must be movement inside the muscle even if it is of such a small degree that it cannot be seen.

Every joint in the body is worked by at least two sets of muscles, one on each side, which become shorter and thicker on contraction and longer and thinner on relaxation. E.g., if the elbow-joint is bent, the biceps (the muscle on the front of the upper arm) is contracted. It will protrude and harden as the elbow is bent more and more. In the position of full flexion of the elbow, the triceps (the muscle on the back of the upper arm) is at its longest and thinnest.

Now, if the arm is stretched out, triceps can be felt to harden and with the elbow fully extended, *it* is at its shortest and broadest while biceps is fully stretched. Relaxation of all muscles is therefore impossible if joints are either fully bent or fully stretched.

Nerve Impulses.—

The brain with the nervous system has been compared to a telephone service. The brain is like the exchange, the central control. The nerves are like the cables, arranged in bundles which go from the exchange to each locality. The nerve-endings in all parts of the body are like the separate instruments used by subscribers, which are dotted about in differing environments over the whole area. There are in-coming and out-going calls at various times to and from subscribers.

Calls from the brain to the nerve-endings produce action in muscle and they are known as motor impulses. Calls from the nerve-endings to the brain are called 'sensory impulses'. They send reports to the central control on what is happening in their immediate locality. They report about temperature and pressure. Pressure, if very great, can cause pain. They also inform headquarters if a part is touched and whether the pressure is hard or soft, smooth or rough.

The Muscular or Kinæsthetic Sense.—

When we think about it, we realize that we are aware of the position of every part of our body, even when the eyes are closed. This is partly because the brain is getting impulses of stretch and movement. In lifting we adapt ourselves to the weight by an assessment of the resistance. The same sense enables us to judge the range and the force of movements by the degree of activity and contraction of muscles.

In athletes, jugglers, and sculptors, for example, the sense is highly developed. Have you ever anticipated lifting a heavy suitcase or a kettle full of water only to find on raising it that it is empty ? It gives one quite a start.

Only when we have learnt to appreciate the feeling of tension in muscles and tendons, through our sensory impulses, can we train ourselves actively to inhibit it by our conscious control. We switch it off, as we would an electric light. We can then relax every part of the body and become un-tensed.

Sometimes, though messages are continuously going to the brain, we are not consciously aware of them. This can apply in many senses but especially to hearing, e.g., people who live near a railway line accustom themselves to the usual noises. They do not notice when the regular trains go by, but they would become aware, immediately, of an unusual noise.

Sensory Check.—Stop reading for a moment or two and listen. You may suddenly realize that there is a clock ticking, yet you had not been hearing it previously. What other noises can you hear ? Had you noticed them before ?

In a similar way, we are going to 'tune in' to some of those messages from our muscles and tendons to our brain which we might not have observed previously.

Position: Sitting, fully supported, with shoes off.

Movements: First, bend the toes on one foot downwards. Can you feel the sensation of tightening on the sole of the foot? The muscles on the *under* surface of the foot are contracting and so it is from that locality that tension is felt.

Next bend all the toes upward. There will be a sensation on the *upper* surface of the foot. Now switch off all activity in the muscles which bend and stretch the toes; let them go quite slack. If they are really relaxed the sensation of tightening will have gone. There is no tension to feel. At the moment the only report that comes through is that the feet are in contact with the object on which they are resting.

Concentrate on the ankles. Bend the foot upwards and there will be a feeling of tightening on the front of the leg, near the shin. Bend the foot downwards and there will be the same sort of feeling in the calf muscles. Let the foot go limp and these slight sensations will have gone.

If these movements are made to the fullest extent, you will feel stretch sensations in skin and tendons on the opposite side to the ones that are contracting. Distinguish between these feelings but try again moving the joint in a smaller range so that stretch is not felt.

Rest one arm comfortably on the arm of a chair, with a cushion if it is not upholstered. Bend the fingers towards the palm of the hand. Where is the tension? Yes, on the palm side of the fingers and hand. Stretch the fingers out straight and it will be felt on the back of the hand and fingers. Let the fingers go loose and, if they are relaxed, they curl up half bent, half stretched.

If you were feeling tension from areas higher up the arm, then you were not *only* moving the fingers. Remember we are teaching ourselves to localize those sensory impulses and we must be careful not to brace up the whole arm as we move the fingers. Try it once more and make sure!

Next, bend the hand downwards from the wrist. Do you feel tension on the under side of forearm and wrist? Now lift the hand upwards and bend the wrist backwards. Has there been a change in the site of the tension? You should be conscious of it on the back of the forearm and wrist.

Having experienced these sensory changes in the limbs, we can progress to learn general relaxation. Once our conscious awareness of tension has been established we can (with practice) inhibit it completely. We are then relaxed.

General Relaxation.—

Full support for every part of the body is essential.

When lying down, a very soft springy bed is not the best medium, because as the body relaxes, the bed sags in the middle and the full support is lost. An unyielding surface is therefore best with a doubled rug or blanket underneath the body.

We can obtain the necessary support in the sitting, prone (forward) lying, half-lying, or back-lying positions. Pillows or cushions are used to accommodate the curves and support the head and limbs wherever they are needed.

All tight clothes should be loosened; the temperature should be comfortably warm (nobody can relax when cold and shivery) and in winter it is sometimes a good idea to cover the body with an extra blanket to protect it from draught.

In pregnancy the left or right side lying position is usually preferred, so let us try that first of all.

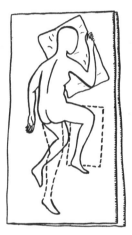

Fig. 9.—Position for relaxation on side. Pillow under upper knee may or may not be needed.

Getting Comfortable.—The diagram above shows how we can modify the basic position to suit our own shape. As pregnancy progresses, the position of the pillows may be adjusted (*Fig.* 9).

One pillow slants downwards and forwards under the head, the upper shoulder, and arm, with the head bent forward slightly. Its purpose is to take up the difference in height between the under shoulder and the side of the face, so that the head is not inclined to either side. If the pillow is too low, there will be pressure on the under shoulder and chest and the head will be bent downwards and sideways, causing discomfort in the neck. If the pillow is too high, then the neck will be stretched on the under-side and discomfort will also be felt within a short time.

Bend the spine forwards enough to reduce the hollow at the waist, placing the upper knee on the floor (or another pillow) in front of the under one.

31

Some people like to have the under leg well bent, others like it almost straight. The length of the thighs, the girth at the level of the hips, and the size of the abdominal bulge will affect our choice of position.

With the under leg straighter the body tends to lie flatter on the support. As the under leg is bent up, the lower trunk and pelvis rotate and pressure is taken off the abdominal wall.

The under arm can be either behind the trunk, down behind the waist, or in front, supported as far as the elbow on the floor, with the forearm across the chest and hand resting on the opposite shoulder.

If after 2 or 3 min. the upper side of the neck begins to ache, it will appear that the pillow is too high. If there is pressure on the under breast or the shoulder is digging into the floor, then the pillow is too low. Do not try to overcome this by placing the shoulder *on* the pillow. Simply push the filling well up against the under shoulder-girdle so that there is no gap and try it again.

On the floor, you might be more comfortable with a pillow under the knee of the upper leg. Test it without and if after a short time you are aware of pressure on the knee or of stretch down the upper thigh, you will probably need one.

Relaxation Training. Step 1.—

When you have found the position which suits you best, settle down to practise. If you have a husband or a friend who will be available to read these instructions out to you later on, so much the better.

1. Breathe low down, easily, and regularly (as taught on page 28 though you may prefer to inspire through the mouth if there is some congestion in the nose). 'Listen' to your own natural rhythm for a few moments:— In—out—in—out.

2. *a.* With the next inward breath, bend the toes up and down slowly (once is enough) and appreciate that feeling of tension as you did in the sitting position previously. Notice also where you feel it.

   b. As you breathe out with a gentle sigh or blow, let the toes go loose.

3. *a.* On breathing in, bend and stretch the ankles slowly. Feel the tension and

   b. On breathing out, let the feet go quite slack.

4. *a.* Breathe in and bend and stretch the knees, just enough to feel the tightening at the back and front of the thigh above the knee.

   b. Breathe out and let the knees go heavy. (If we move the knees too much, we shall get ourselves right out of our comfortable position.)

5. *a.* On breathing in, press the tops of the thighs together and tighten the muscles of the seat and inside of the pelvis, as if trying to control the bowel and the bladder.

   b. On breathing out, let the thighs and buttocks fall apart.

32

6. *a.* On breathing in, draw in the abdominal wall, feel the tightening round the waist and

   b. On breathing out, relax and feel the trunk sinking in the middle until it is completely supported.

7. *a.* On breathing in, stretch the spine, grow taller.

   b. On breathing out, let go and feel the spine recoiling naturally.

8. *a.* On breathing in, shrug the shoulders and

   b. On breathing out, let them droop.

9. *a.* Breathe in, bend and stretch the fingers—think about what you are feeling—and

   b. Breathe out and let them go limp.

10. *a.* Breathe in, bend, and stretch wrists.

    b. Breathe out and allow the hands to flop on the pillow or rug.

11. *a.* Breathe in, bend, and stretch the elbows slightly. (Make sure the hands are still limp when you do it. No need to tense the wrists again, we are only going to move the elbows this time.) Lift the elbows slightly off their support—feel that tightening in the upper arm—and

    b. Breathe out and let the elbows go lax. Be conscious of the *weight* of the arms. They are dragging on the shoulders, dragging down towards the floor.

12. *a.* Breathe in and lift the head up slightly from the pillow—feel the tension in the neck.

    b. Breathe out and let it drop down like a dead weight. (Roll the head a little if you want to and then let go and feel that all the tension has gone from neck and throat.)

    Lastly, we are going to concentrate on the face.

13. *a.* Frown for a second or two, then raise the eyebrows.

    b. Let them go slack.

14. *a.* Close the eyes, open them widely for a moment, as if startled.

    b. Either let them close naturally, or if you prefer to keep them open, feel the lids go loose around the eyes.

15. *a.* Screw up the nose.

    b. Relax it. Feel that all the tension has gone from the side of the nose and cheeks.

16. *a.* Smile, then purse the lips; press the tongue back against the roof of the mouth and suck slightly so that it forms a vacuum.

    b. Let go and feel the mouth and cheeks sagging from the jaws. (This suction action of the tongue against the roof of the mouth will prevent the lower jaw from sagging too much, allowing the mouth to fall open. We do not want this to happen or we shall dribble!)

    When relaxed, the face is quite expressionless.

    Carry on with the regular low-level breathing for about a minute longer and get the feeling of giving yourself up every time you breathe out. From your head right down to your toes you are limp. If a crane were to come along and pick you up with a grip round your middle, you would droop like a rag doll; there would be no resistance.

3   33

The controlled breathing should not be continued for more than 3–4 min. in all. That is approximately the time it will take to go through this routine.

After that, breathe naturally and remain un-tensed for about 15 min. It usually takes beginners about this length of time to reach their maximum of relaxation. Every time it is practised, that maximum will be achieved a little quicker.

The circulation will be slowed and the blood-pressure is likely to be lowered. So when you get up from the lying position, S–T–R–E–T–C–H your arms and legs like an animal and sit up slowly. To do so quickly might cause giddiness; you might even feel faint.

Incidentally the blood-pressure sometimes tends to be raised in pregnancy. Complete relaxation helps to lower the blood-pressure more than an ordinary rest in the chair with the feet up, so the best time to practise it is after the midday meal. At this time the pressure is likely to have reached its highest peak (it will probably be lower in the early morning after a night's sleep). In this way you can reduce your blood-pressure for the second half of the day and you will be revived, and far better company, when your husband comes home in the evening!

If, on the other hand, you have decided to continue with your employment until later in your pregnancy or if you have been out all day doing something unusual, then practise your relaxation as soon as you get home. It would be unwise, after a busy day, to plough straight into cooking or try to rush through household jobs that had not been done earlier.

Practise this general tensing and un-tensing routine daily, trying to recognize the sensation with smaller and smaller movements each day. When you know that you are able to appreciate muscle contraction without movement of joints, you will be ready to progress to *Step* 2.

You may perhaps be thinking, 'Surely all that practice is not really necessary? I shall be able to let go when the time comes, without all that fuss!'

But relaxing when you are comfortable with not a care in the world is quite a different matter from doing it during uterine contractions at the period in labour when most women find conditions uneasy!

With correct method and practice, relaxation becomes automatic in spite of discomfort. If we understand what is happening, mind and body become co-ordinated. It is the same if one is learning to use a typewriter, to drive a car, or to play a musical instrument. The typist trains her sense of touch with eyes away from the instrument; the experienced driver can respond in heavy traffic without conscious control of hands and feet; the concert pianist leaves the written music at home when performing to an audience, yet the sounds seem to flow. At the time he does not consider which fingers are striking the notes on the keyboard, though he has gone through this stage previously in learning the technique of playing.

For the majority, the only way to cultivate the ability to carry relaxation into full effect at the right time during labour is through practice and progression and in this way you will help yourself through pregnancy as well.

When you think you have trained yourself to relax completely ask your husband or friend to test you by lifting your hand off the pillow. The elbow should still hang down towards its support and the hand should flop down again on to the pillow when dropped. If the elbow is lifted by somebody else, the hand should still drop downwards. It should be possible for them to move your arm up, down, and sideways without any resistance from you. When the uplifting pressure is taken away, the arm should not stay in mid-air but drop naturally, wherever it is. This is controlled inhibition of muscular tension and it demands your concentration to *keep* your muscles in this state of relaxation.

Relaxation Training. Step 2.—

No bending or stretching movements are now required, since you will be aware of tension, if it is present, even without apparent movement. You have passed the initial stage and can appreciate the difference between a contracted and a relaxed muscle.

Start off by getting comfortably supported on your left or right side in the position you have found suits you best.

1. Begin doing the easy, regular low-level breathing as before. 'Listen' to the natural rhythm and sigh or blow gently as you breathe out.
2. *a.* With the next breath in, concentrate on the toes (but don't move them).
   b. As you breathe out, let them go loose.
3. *a.* As you breathe in, think about the ankles.
   b. On breathing out, let the feet go slack.
4. *a.* Breathe in . . . think about knees.
   b. Breathe out . . . let the legs go heavy.
5. *a.* Breathe in . . . think about thighs, buttocks and inside the pelvis.
   b. Breathe out . . . let the thighs and buttocks fall apart.

Continue in this way, concentrating on each area in turn with an ingoing breath, and letting go with a sigh, until every part of the legs, body, upper limbs, neck, and face is relaxed. You may feel that you are floating or resting on cotton-wool.

Another day, try going through the same routine on your back, half-lying supported with pillows (*Fig.* 10 A) or lying (*Fig.* 10 B). Lying flat on the spine sometimes causes backache. If so, go back to the side-lying and try to keep the weight of the baby away from the spine.

Remember that neither we nor our babies are all exactly the same shape, and in the latter part of pregnancy the babies are moving around and exercising themselves fairly frequently. It is possible then that you might prefer lying on your back at one time and on your side at another. You will find that if you are restless at night, relaxation with easy regular breathing will help you to get off to sleep.

Sometimes relax in an arm-chair, fully supported (*see Fig. 5 C*, p. 21). If you have been sitting at a table writing or working, lean over the table for a short spell and rest the head on the hands or wrists. Let the shoulders, arms, and body slacken and thighs fall apart (*Fig.* 10 C).

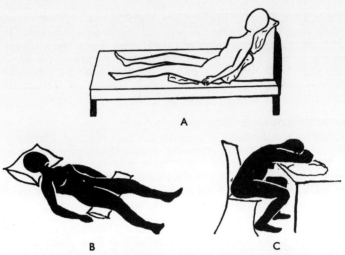

Fig. 10.—A, Relaxation in half-lying position; B, Relaxation in lying position; C, Relaxation in sitting position.

All of these positions may be helpful to you in labour, so it is beneficial to get accustomed to them.

You will soon find that the easy regular breathing, with a gentle sigh or blow on expiration, has become the key to relaxation. As you do it, you will relax automatically.

Breathing Control for the First Stage of Labour.—

Every woman has her own natural breathing rhythm and we do not want to interfere with it. Nevertheless you will find that as the contractions become stronger and last a little longer the chest wall will expand on a higher level and breathing will quicken towards and over the crest. It then slows down to the normal tranquil pace and depth.

The same thing would happen if you climbed a flight of stairs and came straight back down again; but your breathing would speed up more if the stairway was steeper and higher than if the risers were arranged to give an easier gradient. There is a similar wave-like pattern of ascents, crests, and descents running through the first stage of labour but nobody knows beforehand what sort of swell they will have to cope with. We should accept these natural forces which Nature provides to help us, one way or another, and adapt our breathing to them.

Breathing Adaptation Exercise.—

Position: Sitting or lying, back and head fully supported.

1. Easy regular low-level breathing (which has already been mentioned with 'Relaxation').
2. Slightly accelerated middle-level breathing. Feel the ribs rising sideways gently with the ingoing breaths and falling again with the *outgoing* ones. Concentrate on relaxing the chest, shoulders, 'tummy' and back with each expiration.
3. Slightly faster higher level breathing. Become aware of your breast-bone (where a pendant would rest) moving up and down gently as you breathe in and out. Make the soft blowing noises you would hear yourself making if you had run up a flight of stairs. Again, remember to slacken as you breathe OUT.

Make the changeover from (1) to (2) and (2) to (3) smoothly. Change down again and practise with relaxation in all the positions which you might use in labour, i.e., sitting, lying on the side, and half-lying on the back, but remember that when you are in labour it will be much easier, because you will have both your natural inclinations and your medical and midwifery attendants to guide you.

Relaxation Training. Step 3. Selective Relaxation.—
This is to train your ability to *maintain* a state of relaxation everywhere else in your body, while one muscle (or group of muscles) is contracting strongly. The idea is that muscle contractions in the arms (which are controlled by your will) simulate the contractions of the uterus (which is *not* controlled by the will).

It should be practised before the birth only, to train your co-ordination.

You will find that you need to concentrate more than in the previous exercises but that is all to the good. Part of the object of the exercise is to develop your powers of concentration.

After being contracted strongly for about three-quarters of a minute, muscles begins to ache because fatigue products have collected and are pressing on nerve-endings. This is exactly what happens during contractions of the uterus and then between them blood flows in bringing fresh oxygen supplies and the 'ash' is carried away.

Labour can seem harsh and fatiguing towards the end of the first stage where the natural forces seem to build up with unrelenting fervour. The discipline will help you to remain at ease as conditions get more difficult, by focusing your attention on your breathing rhythm and the complete relaxation of every other controllable part of your body.

Position: Lying, with a round object (ball, apple, or orange) in your left hand, pillows supporting back, shoulders, head, and another under thighs.

Imagine a Uterine Contraction starting Now.—At the same time:—

Contract the left hand and fore-arm and squeeze on the round object. Go on contracting and squeezing harder and harder for about 15 seconds; then slowly release it for 15 seconds.	Breathe in, breathe out, and keep up the easy, regular low-level breathing, while maintaining every other part of your body in a state of complete relaxation, until the left arm and hand have stopped contracting.

Repeat the next day with the round object in the right hand. Then you will contract the right arm and maintain relaxation in the left arm and every other part of the body, while breathing easily and regularly for about 30 seconds.

Next, link it up with the 'Breathing Adaptation Exercise' but read Chapter IV, 'The Application—During Birth', before trying it out.

1. 30 seconds: As above.
2. 45 seconds: Start with easy regular low-level breathing as you begin to squeeze the ball. After about 15 seconds change to middle-level slightly accelerated breathing. Continue for about 15 seconds (over crest) and then slow down to previous pace and depth, gradually releasing ball.
3. 1 minute: Start to squeeze and breathe calmly, low down. After a few seconds, rise to middle level (slightly accelerated) and continue until you become aware of movement in the upper chest —squeezing harder all the time with one arm and relaxing everywhere else. Keep it up over the 'crest' for about 20 seconds and then slow down again smoothly to normal speed and level for another 20 seconds, while your grip on the ball is reduced.

The Final Progression in Relaxation Training. Step 4.—

When you have mastered *Steps* 1, 2, and 3, have someone else— your husband, a relative, or friend—grip your leg with their thumbs and fingers to the point where it hurts. This enables them to assess how much squeezing you can take. Some people are much more sensitive than others.

N.B.—If you have any signs of varicose veins in the legs, then have them put the pressure on an arm near the elbow, instead.

They should be able to find a spot where increasing force becomes very uncomfortable. If they seem unable to find a painful area, a pinching action on the thigh may do the trick!

You are now going to train yourself to keep tension 'switched off' while feelings of pressure—which you cannot control by your own will —build up and diminish.

Position: Lying on back or side, comfortably supported.

1. Get that someone to increase the pressure gradually for about 20 seconds—but not to the limit of your endurance—then decrease it for another 20 seconds.

   While this is going on, imagine it as a contraction of the uterus (no, it will not feel exactly like this but similar, perhaps). Switch off tension as soon as the pressurizing starts and *think* your way over it. *Stay* relaxed, particularly in 'tummy', pelvic floor, thighs, back, chest, and shoulders. Listen to the rhythm of your outgoing breaths—consciously slump with each one until the pressure has gone. (About 40 seconds in all.)
2. Progress to 25 seconds going up. When gripping starts, relax completely. With rather more pressure, slightly accelerate breathing and change smoothly to middle level. Imagine floating over the

crest while still more force is being exerted for about 10 seconds. Then down the other side for 25 seconds—pressure decreasing, breathing decelerating.

At the end, take a big, deep breath (which is natural after a satisfying effort) and sigh, thinking 'one more behind and one less in front'. (About 1 minute in all.)

3. Progress to 30 seconds going up. As pressure starts, 'switch off' tension—think about those special muscle groups in the same order—adapt breathing as the pressure increases and go through middle level to higher level, still keeping relaxed. Stay on top riding the crest of the wave while being subjected to maximum pressure lasting for about 20 seconds, breathing almost effortlessly, absolutely relaxed. Down again as the force subsides, listening to the slowing rhythm of breathing. A big deep breath and sigh at the end. (Just over 1¼ minutes in all.)

3.—GENERAL EXERCISES BEFORE BIRTH

A busy woman does not want or need a long scheme of exercises to perform daily. For the first four months of pregnancy, follow the methods of self-instruction in the preceding sections. Teach yourself to adopt, automatically, a position for all parts of the body, in which fatigue is cut down to the minimum, movement is easiest, and work is safest (by elimination of strain), and learn to relax completely.

From four months onward, certain exercises will be helpful:—

1. To improve tone and elasticity of muscles.
2. To promote ease of movement in spinal and pelvic joints, while maintaining maximum stability.
3. To aid the circulation, particularly in the feet, legs, and pelvis.

Plan your campaign towards every part of your body which might prove a weak spot under increased stress.

Exercise 1.—*For strengthening the Feet and preventing Congestion in the Circulation of Blood in the Lower Limbs.*

Position: Sit down comfortably with the back supported against the head of the bed or a wall; legs straight.

Movements:

a. Bend and stretch the ankles 6 times.

b. Pretend that you are sitting on a sandy beach and gather imaginary sand into little heaps between your feet, with circling movements of ankles.

Repeat 6–12 times, increasing gradually.

Exercise 2.—*For Pelvic Floor Control, Check your Undercarriage.*

The muscles of the pelvic floor form a double hammock across the bony outlet of the pelvis, to support the bladder, the uterus, and the rectum (lower part of the bowel). They are divided in midline to allow the urethra (bladder outlet), vagina, and anus (bowel outlet) to pass through, and there are U-shaped slings, like elasticized pyjama cords,

39

giving extra support to these channels (*Fig.* 11). Towards the end of pregnancy, they become softened and their elasticity is increased. During the second stage of labour, they have a part to play in rotating the baby and directing it downwards and forwards underneath the arch

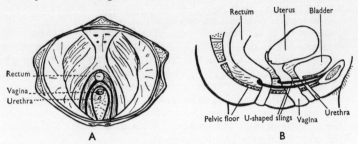

Fig. 11.—A, The pelvic floor muscles from above; B, The pelvic floor muscles from the right, showing the U-shaped slings supporting the rectum, vagina, and urethra.

of bone in the front of the pelvis; then they part in midline and when completely relaxed, the edges are drawn up easily over the oncoming head.

You have contracted your pelvic floor muscles on many occasions in your life when trying to control a full bladder or rectum. When you have done this, the edges of the muscle in midline have been drawn closer together and the whole sling of muscle has been lifted slightly and tightened up to give additional support where necessary.

This is exactly the action that some women do, unwittingly, a short time before their baby is born. It narrows the aperture, makes the birth more difficult for mother and child, and perhaps even more important, puts a far greater and quite unnecessary strain on the muscle tissue of the pelvic floor. A strained muscle takes some time to recover its full strength. We need to have good tone and control of these muscles during birth, with the ability to stretch easily and recoil quickly afterwards. Localized exercises can help us to achieve such a state.

Pelvic Floor Contraction and Relaxation.

Position: Sitting on a low stool or chair with knees apart, trunk leaning forward and elbows resting on knees (*Fig.* 12 A).

Movements:

1. Contract as if to control the bowel—concentrate as you do it, and sense that you are drawing up inside, and not 'cheating' by contracting the buttocks only—then relax completely. This action should produce an obvious feeling of tension in the fibres of muscle towards the back of the pelvic floor, as the anus is lifted and squeezed.

    Repeat the movement twice more—3 times in all—with smooth wave-like contraction and relaxation.

2. Contract as if to control the bladder. Do not press the thighs together. Then relax completely. This action should produce a feeling of tension inside, more to the front of the pelvic floor as, with a similar compressing action on the vagina and urethra, both these passages are crowded towards the front of the pelvis. Concentrate as you repeat it twice more, and feel the *forward* pull.

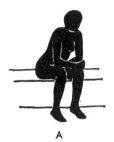 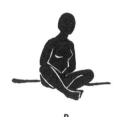

A   B

Fig. 12.—Position for pelvic floor movements. A, Sitting with elbows on parted knees; B, Sitting, back supported, knees bent and outwardly rotated, soles of feet together.

3. Contract first the back fibres (as for bowel control), then the front fibres (as for bladder control), and finally behave as if you were trying to draw air inside the vagina. You should sense a definite lift of the whole pelvic floor. Follow with relaxation and repeat *twice* more. Be aware of the slight difference in sensation as each part of the muscle is tensed and when you let go, feel your undersling slacken and descend.

At first you may be conscious of very little happening, and the first, second, and third types of contraction may seem very much the same to you. With practice you will become more proficient.

N.B.—The tempo is important. Before birth the contraction and relaxation of the pelvic floor muscles should be wave-like, rhythmically drawing them up and straightway down again. In this way the elasticity of muscle can be improved.

When you have mastered the movement sitting on a chair, you can do it in:—

Alternative Positions:
1. Side lying, as for relaxation.
2. Sitting on the bed or floor, with back supported, knees and hips well bent up, soles of feet together, knees apart (*Fig.* 12 B).

Train yourself to appreciate the difference in the action and movement of the pelvic floor muscles when:—

1. Trying to pass a motion—the direction of pressure is downwards and *backwards*.
2. Trying to prevent bowel evacuation—the back of the pelvic floor is lifted and the anus is squeezed.

3. Trying to empty the bladder—the direction of pressure is downwards and *forwards*; the same course, in fact, as a baby takes when being born.
4. Trying to prevent leakage from the bladder—the vagina and urethra are drawn *forwards* and upwards towards the front of the pelvis and compressed with a gentle nut-cracker action.

Exercises 3, 4, and 5.—*To Strengthen the Suspension of the Pelvis and the Three-way-stretch Girdle of Muscle which supports the Baby and Abdominal Organs.*

There are three basic movements, each of which should be performed daily and repeated not more than 6 times (less if you feel that you have had enough), bearing in mind that the correct pelvic tilt is the 'cornerstone', so to speak, on which sound posture is built. These pelvic movements will help you to develop an automatic postural sense not only in standing, but in any position in which the body is required to rest, move, or work.

Exercise 3.—For the Straight Front Abdominal Muscles (which tilt the front of the pelvis up towards the ribs), working with the Muscles of the Seat (which pull the back of it downwards).

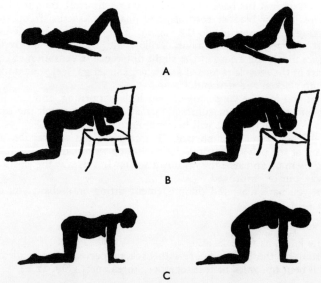

Fig. 13.—Pelvic uptilting: A, Lying with knees bent; B, Prone kneeling over chair; C, Prone kneeling on bed or floor.

Positions:
1. Standing with back against a wall, feet slightly apart and one foot-length away from the wall, or
2. Lying on the back with knees bent up and slightly apart (*Fig.* 13 A).

42

Movements:

1. Press the waist against the wall or the floor and draw the pelvis up in front towards the ribs.
2. Relax and let the spine return to its natural hollow at waist level.

The following starting positions will relieve backache and are more beneficial after 6 months of pregnancy, particularly when, of necessity, you have been standing for some time.

They will also help the abdominal organs to fall into their correct places (they are suspended from the spine) and relieve congestion in the pelvis:—

Alternative positions:

1. Kneeling with forearms resting on the seat of a chair; forehead may rest on hands, trunk prone (*Fig.* 13 B).
2. Prone kneeling on bed or floor (*Fig.* 13 C).

Movements:

1. Draw the pelvis up in front, rounding the waist and tucking the seat down and underneath.
2. Relax, allowing the waist to hollow again, naturally.

Exercise 4.—For the Straight Muscles at the Side of the Waist, which tilt the Pelvis towards the Ribs on the same side, causing Shrugging of the Hips and Apparent Shortening of One Leg.

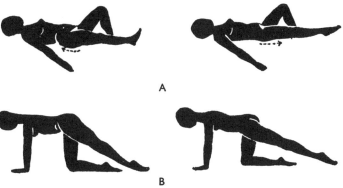

A

B

Fig. 14.—A, Hip shrugging, lying on back, one knee bent; B, Prone kneeling, one leg extended.

Positions:

1. Lying on back with one knee bent and one straight (*Fig.* 14 A), or
2. Kneeling (forearms may rest on the seat of a chair), one leg stretched out straight backwards, with toes touching floor (*Fig.* 14 B).

43

Movements:

1. Draw the hip of the straight leg up towards the ribs on the same side (leg seems shorter).
2. Press it down again (leg seems longer). Repeat 6 times with each leg.

N.B.—Pelvic and abdominal movements should be performed smoothly, and rhythmically. Then they have an uplifting effect without straining.

Exercise 5.—For the Oblique Muscles which cross over from Ribs to Pelvis on the opposite side and on contraction cause a twisting movement of the Pelvis.

Position: Standing with trunk bent forward, arms reaching straight ahead to grasp the back of a firm chair, cooker, or shelf.

Movements:

1. Put all your weight on the right leg.
2. Swing the left leg to the back and then around smoothly to the left side, then front and across to the right in a big wide circle. Pelvis should turn to the limit (left hip forward) while arms hold the support throughout the movement.
3. Uncoil by swinging the left leg around the 'maypole' in the opposite direction—to the front, left side, back, and across to the limit on the right, turning the hips as far as they will go (right hip forward).

    Repeat 4–6 times in both directions. Rest for half a minute and then do it standing on the left leg. (*Fig.* 15.)

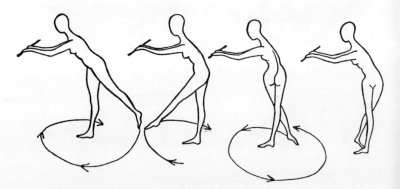

Fig. 15.—Pelvic rotation. Standing. Reaching forward and grasping support.

The Bustline.—
Motherhood actually improves most figures *if* the supportive tissues are not overstrained.

The cells in the breasts which develop and enlarge in pregnancy are covered by protective fatty tissue and completely enclosed in what is known as 'connective tissue'. It allows for a certain amount of expansion but is strong and semi-transparent, looking rather like a plastic bag.

There is no muscle tissue in the breast itself but the 'plastic containers' are continued up to the breast-bones, collar-bones, and shoulders and they are attached very firmly over most of the surfaces of the pectoral muscles (which you can feel in front of your armpits). These strong, elastic, fan-shaped muscles suspend the bosoms from the bones in the shoulder area.

A well-fitting 'bra' made like two gentle hammocks takes a lot of the strain off the elastic fibres and prevents them getting overstretched. When a 'bra' is too large or fails to support properly—or worse, when one is not worn at all—the pull of gravity plays havoc with the muscle fibres and the 'plastic bag' begins to droop. You know how inefficient worn-out elastic is!

Lack of support spoils the shape—not breast-feeding!

If you have had children before and your line is not what it was, do not believe the pessimists who say that it is too late to do any good. You can! Improve the tone *before* having this baby and work hard at the following exercises now and afterwards.

Exercise 6.—*To strengthen and tone up the Chest Muscles.*

Position: Sitting or standing upright. Cross the arms on shoulder level and grasp the opposite arms just above or below the elbows on the inside (*Fig.* 16).

Fig. 16.—Pectoral exercise.

Movements: Press the hands hard towards the upper arms and try to force the elbows across and apart. Give firm movements followed by relaxation. Do them in quick succession, about one press every second.

Repeat 10–20 times.

Let the arms drop down to the sides and relax for a few moments. Then:—

Position: Sitting or standing arms crossed as before.

Movements: Stretch *forward* with the elbows, reaching out as far as possible and follow with relaxation at the same tempo.

N.B.—In both these exercises the elbows must be kept at shoulder level.

45

Exercise 7.—*Squatting.*

In this position of rest, which we all used until stools and chairs were thought of, the pelvis is at its widest capacity.

Modified squatting positions, in lying, side lying, and half lying, are used in the second stage of labour, and if they are adopted with the trunk upright for lifting, gardening, and cleaning (*see Fig.* 6 E, F, page 23), the effect will be:—

1. To increase suppleness.
2. To accustom yourself beforehand to a position which may be required of you, with slight changes, in labour.
3. To get the jobs done with minimal strain on the back.

Position a: Hold on to a firm support (e.g., the side of the bath or the kitchen sink) with feet straight, about 1 ft. apart.

Movement: Keeping the heels flat on the floor bend the hips and knees and push the thighs comfortably apart. Go down slowly, through a wicket-keeper's position, until the body is at rest with knees and hips fully bent and a rounded back. Relax except for the hands which are holding on. Come up again by pressing feet on the floor and straightening the knees and hips (*Fig.* 17 A).

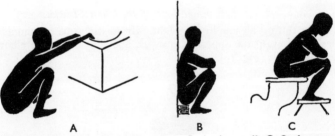

Fig. 17.—Squatting: A, Holding bath; B, Against wall; C, On lavatory.

Position b: Stand with the back to a wall with feet straight, about 6 in. in front of it and 6–12 in. apart.

Movement: Leaning against the wall, slide the back gently down until the seat comes to rest on small books stacked about 6 inches high. Relax in this position for a few moments and then rise by pushing feet against the floor and contracting the thigh muscles (*Fig.* 17 B).

Position c: Use the squatting position to aid expulsion from the pelvis. It is the natural one and it assists movement of the bowel and excretion without straining. Pressure from the thighs against the abdominal wall, above the groin, will help to start movement— at the customary time—within a minute or two. Place a stool or box in front of the lavatory seat and put the feet on it with knees comfortably apart, and lean well forward so that the thighs are in contact with the abdominal wall on either side (*Fig.* 17 C).

46

Notes concerning Exercises.—

Seven exercises have been suggested for you, but the starting positions are numerous. Use only one of these basic positions at any one time—variety is the spice of life—and though it may suit you to go through all of them in one go, the exercises can sometimes be more effective if they are fitted in little by little with the everyday round.

Always stop short if feeling tired, and relax completely for a few moments before performing another exercise or continuing with the chores.

These movements will also be the basis of the scheme of exercises for restoration to full activity and well-being after birth. When they have been practised pre-natally, even though muscle stretching takes place and some degree of tone is lost temporarily, it is regained more quickly. Faulty postural habits which undermine or retard total restoration are not allowed to develop.

Internal Examinations.—When the doctor or midwife prepares to make an internal examination, either in pregnancy or in labour, relax the pelvic floor and abdominal muscles completely and breathe easily and regularly (as in BREATHING EXERCISE, p. 28) while it is being done. They will find it very much easier to make their investigation.

Warning.—

Avoid over-accentuation of the hollow-back position, both during pregnancy, while the pelvic and sacro-iliac joints are lax, and after birth, until they have tightened up again—a process which may take from 3 to 6 months.

Orthopædic specialists say that arching the spine backwards from the waist to the limit of movement may cause overstretching of the ligaments at those joints and that, by maintaining such movement after the birth of a baby, they are not permitted to shrink, spontaneously, to their pre-pregnant state of stability. This can be the cause of chronic backache.

Avoid over-strong abdominal work until you have had your post-natal check-up by your doctor, 6 weeks after the baby is born.

Do not perform exercises which are strenuous enough to make you hold your breath. If this happens the diaphragm is pushed down and there is a forward and downward thrust of the abdominal contents. This may cause the straight front abdominal muscles to part in the midline.

If you are lying on your back and you lift both legs or raise your trunk up to a sitting position, towards the end of pregnancy, it may have just this effect. The front abdominal muscles bow forward and sometimes separate, while the intestines (and the baby) are forced forward and downwards through the gaps in the 'tummy' wall and pelvic floor.

Similarly, when taking a bath, bulging may be observed when changing from sitting to lying in the water.

It is wise not to allow this additional stress. Roll over sideways on getting up (e.g., out of bed) and push the trunk upwards by using the palms of the hands and the arms.

In the bath, assist yourself to sit up by using the hands and arms to pull or push up.

IV. THE APPLICATION—DURING BIRTH

WHEN AND HOW TO ASSIST YOURSELF, FROM THE END OF PREGNANCY TO THE END OF LABOUR

At about 8 months, the baby is usually higher in the abdominal cavity than at any time during pregnancy. The mother's intestines and stomach are compressed and even the bases of her lungs have less room to expand. At this time it is usual to get more breathless on going upstairs, and indigestion is common after meals. It may be quite a feat to put on stockings and shoes in the usual way. To do this more easily, sit down, cross the legs and rest one ankle across the other knee. Now you can draw the foot up close enough to reach the toes.

Lightening.—When you come to the last weeks of pregnancy, you will feel your abdomen hardening and tightening. This is due to muscular contractions of the uterus, which can be felt through the abdominal wall. These contractions in the upper part of the uterus are simply pushing the baby gently down into the brim of the pelvic basin (the fluid takes the pressure, not the baby).

'Lightening', as it is called, happens sometimes slowly and sometimes quickly. There is no definite rule as to when it should occur, but afterwards your doctor or midwife may comment that the baby's head is 'engaged', or 'down in the brim'.

Some women mistake these contractions for the onset of labour, and hurry off to hospital, or nursing home, if that is where they have booked to have their babies, and on arrival, maybe before, contractions stop.

It is rather frustrating to imagine that you will have the baby by to-morrow, only to be told that you are not in labour! So it will be as well to know that the contractions which push the baby down into the pelvis beforehand are not as a rule, regular. Though occasionally they are regular for a short time, they peter out and stop. Sometimes they occur during the night and do not even break one's sleep.

When this has occurred, you will be less breathless, because there will be more room to breathe deeply. You will then be able to put on shoes and stockings with comparative ease.

Labour.—

Labour is the effort of the female body to expel the reproduced young. It entails muscle work, most of which is quite outside the conscious control, and some of which is controlled by the will. There are three stages:—

First Stage—The thinning and opening up of the cervix to full dilatation.

Second Stage—The expulsion from the uterus, and birth of the baby.

Third Stage—The separation and expulsion of the placenta (afterbirth), membranes, and the rest of the cord.

48

The Onset of Labour.—

The Show.—At some time, possibly in early labour, due to the movement in the 'bottle-neck' (cervix), the mucus plug is loosened and the 'stopper' comes away. It is a jelly-like substance, sometimes pinkish or streaked with blood, and this is known as the 'show'.

Contractions.—There are numerous sensations that may be felt during contractions. Women vary greatly in this, and having produced a family of three or four, one might say that the early sensations were different in character with the birth of each child.

More commonly, the contractions are not at first very strong, last only about half a minute, and they may be felt as waves of any of the following:—

1. Dull backache.
2. A dragging-down sensation low in the front of the abdomen, 'like a period pain'.
3. A colicky disturbance—the sort of discomfort that is felt after eating green apples, plums, or taking a dose of purgative.
4. A feeling of downward pressure, starting at the waist and pressing down toward the groin.
5. A combination of backache and 'tummy-ache'—it may start at the back and work round to the front, or start in the front and radiate to the back.
6. The thighs or hips may ache.

When the pressure is increased to any extent in the hollow abdominal organs (e.g., wind in the stomach or intestines) it usually produces perceptible changes in sensation. The uterus is no exception.

Childbirth without sensory changes usually means childbirth without warning! Is this what we want? To have our babies unexpectedly in places we would not choose? Better surely to feel the natural signals which seem to say: 'You're going to have this baby. Get organized. Make for a place of safety.' Nearly every woman has plenty of time to do all she needs to do before she settles down to welcome her baby.

Sometimes there is uncertainty as to whether labour is beginning, or whether the sensations are the result of something unusual recently eaten—understandable, perhaps, since there may be a desire to empty the bowel at an unusual time. However, if the uterus is contracting, it can be felt through the abdominal wall, hardening for a short time and softening again when the contraction has passed.

At first the contractions may last anything from a few seconds up to about a minute, usually with a definite rhythm, once labour is established, but the intervals vary considerably. Commonly they start at about 20–30-minute intervals and the forces become gradually closer and stronger, until by the end of the first stage they may be repeated every 2–3 min.

Some women start with the contractions coming as far apart as 40–60 min., and some, equally normally, start with them coming as closely as 5 or even 3 min. apart.

None of us has the slightest control over the speed with which these contractions occur, or over their power. In some cases the uterus has a rest and contractions cease altogether for a period and then start up again. We must just take childbirth as it comes and give ourselves up to it entirely. Therefore it should not be regarded as something to be proud of to have a baby quickly. The slower, smoother labours can be perfect from everybody's viewpoint, except perhaps the waiting husband's!

It would be a mistake to anticipate labour lasting any specific length of time, but with a first baby, the stage of dilatation can be expected to last between twelve and twenty-four hours, and the expulsive stage between one and two hours. Remember, though, that there have been completely satisfactory labours which have lasted more and less than the average in both first and second stages.

Rupture of the Membranes (or breaking of the bag of waters).—
This is the filmy, thin, but very strong sac containing the fluid or liquor. Though this more commonly happens towards the end of the first stage or the beginning of the second stage, it can happen quite normally at any time during either stage, and sometimes even before rhythmic contractions are felt at all. Often it is just a trickle, and sometimes, if the bag breaks low down, there is a sudden gush and all the water in front of the baby comes away. The baby's head then fits snugly into the soft cervix like a solid rubber ball plugging a wash basin, and the fluid behind is retained.

If your membranes rupture prior to feeling definite contractions, you will be required to contact your doctor, midwife, or hospital. Ask them about this.

On some occasions the doctor may consider it helpful for the membranes to be ruptured artificially either before or during labour.

Procedure.—Some hospitals and nursing homes advise their patients to stay quietly at home carrying on as usual by night or day until the contractions have narrowed down to 15 (some say 10)-minute intervals, unless the membranes have ruptured. Others advise entering as soon as contractions become regular, whatever the intervals. Obviously, distance would make a difference if travelling time has to be considered, so on this point, too, consult your doctor or midwife.

During the early part of labour, it is much better to be occupied in the day-time whether at home or not. Contractions are noticed less when there is something else to think about, and quite a large part of the first stage may be spent in carrying on light housework, cooking, sewing, or some activity which absorbs the interest.

At night it is important to get as much sleep as possible in early labour, otherwise the patient may be very tired by the time the most concentrated muscular effort is required. If labour starts in the evening, you would probably be advised to settle down in the place where the baby is to be born, before bed-time, secure in the knowledge that you are on the spot, and if the baby *does* arrive before morning you will be awakened!

Always report by telephone or send a message, unless this is impossible, before going into hospital or nursing home. You should feel free to inquire of doctor or midwife, also, if at any time you have doubts connected with the birth.

If your baby is going to be born at home, you should have met your midwife beforehand, or have been told when to get in touch with her.

Routine Toilet and Observation.—

At some time during the first stage, usually soon after admittance to hospital, the patient is made ready for labour. This may involve a bath—it is most comforting to wallow in warm water, though this may not be permitted if the membranes have ruptured—an enema, and shaving of the pubic hair. The enema is to clear the rectum, so that there is more room at the back of the pelvis and you are advised to empty the bladder fairly frequently, so that there is more available space in the front as well. Tell your midwife if at any time you are unable to do this.

The urine may be tested and pulse and blood-pressure checked. The baby's heart-beat is noted and an assessment is made by internal examination (either vaginal or rectal) of how much, if any, dilatation of the cervix has taken place.

Alternative Positions to adopt during Contractions.—Except at night, few women wish to lie down in the early first stage. If the trunk is upright, the pull of gravity can assist the fœtus down into the pelvic basin. During the day, women usually prefer not to recline until the baby is well down into the pelvis.

Whether you are standing, sitting, or lying, round the spine by bending forwards from the waist during first stage contractions. This position widens the pelvic inlet by swivel action. The spine moves backwards slightly at the sacro-iliac joints, and there is reduced pressure on sacral nerves, and therefore less discomfort. *N.B.*: Never hollow the spine by leaning backwards in a deep arm-chair. The position narrows the pelvic inlet and usually adds to the discomfort.

Let yourself go, in whichever position you have chosen, leaning forward, and begin doing the easy regular low-level breathing. Focus your attention on keeping relaxed, particularly, the abdominal and pelvic floor muscles, the back, shoulder and seat muscles, and on letting the thighs droop apart. Maintain the smooth rhythmical respirations so long as they last. Between contractions, carry on reading, sewing, knitting, solving puzzles, listening to the radio, playing cards, watching television, talking, or whatever other quiet pursuit you have chosen to do, until you feel that you want to lie down. This does not mean that the cervix has dilated any particular amount, but it usually means that the baby is well down in the pelvic basin. Some women want to recline fairly early in the first stage and others prefer to keep upright until the cervix is almost fully dilated. There are occasions when patients are advised by their attendants that it is necessary to lie down and rest, but usually when recumbency is desirable to the patient it is the right time for her to lie down.

Relaxation.—Begin relaxing fully during contractions now, lying either on the side or on the back propped up with pillows, wedge, or backrest, with the easy regular low-level breathing as practised previously. Listen to your breathing rhythm so long as each contraction lasts—it will have a soothing effect on you—and let your whole body sink into the bed. If the contractions are strong you will automatically adjust your breathing to middle-level respirations and the rhythm will quicken towards the crest and slow down after it has passed. Towards the end you will once again be breathing as you were at the beginning of the contraction.

Each contraction is like a wave. Imagine them as the waves of the sea. You have gone out in a boat in summertime and the engine has failed. You realize that there is no need to row and exhaust yourself; the harbour is near and the tide is steadily, smoothly, carrying you towards it. Each wave brings the shore nearer as you recline in the boat, giving yourself up to the buoyant drift of the sea, and float towards it.

The difference is, though, that as you get nearer to the end of the first stage, the waves get stronger and heavier—more like mid-channel surges, or possibly Atlantic or Pacific rollers—steeply up, almost flat on top, for a sustained period and then steeply down again.

The Last Part of the First Stage.—Remember that it is important to *concentrate* on remaining relaxed—thinking your orders to your body.

Some people seem to be able to direct their thoughts better with their eyes closed and others with them open, fixed on something in the room.

Meet the waves in the right way and you will keep your balance.

There may be recognizable indications that the second stage is not very far ahead—like buoys to guide you—during the last part of the first stage.

1. *A reflex jerk* as the diaphragm involuntarily contracts and compresses the abdominal contents. When this occurs, it may cause a catch in the breath, a belch, a hiccough, or a grunt. It is not indigestion, but part of the normal pattern of labour!

   Since the stomach lies just underneath the diaphragm on the left side, this sudden jerk against it can make the contents regurgitate. It is not unusual to be sick at this point, but even this can be encouraging to a woman who understands what is happening.

2. *Breathing changes*: After the diaphragm 'twitches', there is a natural inability to relax the abdominal muscles or to breathe low down with the bases of the lungs. Continue quietly relaxing the rest of the body during contractions, and breathing easily and regularly with the middle and upper part of the chest. Expand the ribs sideways and lift the breast-bone as you breathe in—as if you were slightly out of breath—and sigh or blow softly as you breathe out.

3. *Sacral nerve pressure*: There may be pressure during contractions on the nerves on the inside of the pelvis. This is usually greatest during the last part of the first stage, and the last $\frac{1}{5}$ of dilatation is considered by the majority of women to be the most trying part of

52

labour. If the pressure is on a nerve which supplies the lower limbs, it might cause quivering of the legs for a short time, or it might, perhaps, cause a toothachey sort of pain in the buttocks or down the legs. Let your legs go slack; you can be sure it will not last long.

You will ride the resulting discomfort or pain, should it occur, if you think of it in the right way, as simple pressure. *There are absolutely no sensations of internal stretching as the cervix opens up.*

At this time you may need to speed up your breathing still more and think about keeping the chest movement high—well away from the uterus.

On the other hand you may find that the middle level is right for you. You might at no time—not even at the end of the first stage—want to go higher.

One should neither overbreathe nor underbreathe. Whatever you do, it should be rhythmical and smooth with a little more emphasis on the relaxed *expiration*—not forced—and it should feel natural.

It is commonest for women at this stage to feel strong backache during contractions, or there may be pain referred to the front of the abdomen (pressure on a nerve at one place can cause discomfort to be felt somewhere else along the course of the nerve). The prepared patient takes this in her stride, knowing that the trying phase will soon be over and that when the second stage has begun, the direction of power will be downward and forward, with the sacral nerve pressure finished and done with!

Incidentally, that backache is usually greatly eased by counter-pressure on the outside of the sacrum. Massage with a flat hand pressed firmly against the base of the spine can be extremely comforting. Some husbands can be a strong support at this time and their presence may be appreciated if they understand the birth process and help to create an atmosphere of calm, with quiet encouragement.

Relief of Pain.—

Since the days of Queen Victoria, when women in childbirth were first given relief from pain in the form of anæsthetic, expectant mothers have tended to expect either this or some form of dope to ease . . . well, they knew not quite what. People said it was a painful business and one would certainly imagine that it must be! Yet nobody described the discomfort.

Facing an unknown situation usually stimulates the imagination and produces a state of tension. It is not surprising that some women still feel like the famous journalist who recently wrote in one of our national newspapers, "Give me as much anæsthetic as I can get, and when I come round I shall have had the baby and the room will be full of flowers!"

The attitude is changing. Who is better than the woman in labour herself to judge whether relief from pain is necessary? Relief should be available when the time comes and it would be folly to try to do without it, in the competitive sense, yet some women do in fact decline it when it is offered, and a few do not find any part of labour painful.

53

There are some who wish to experience the whole birth with senses undulled. If they are *not* feeling pain, they may resent drugs, which make them feel even slightly dopey, being given as a routine without any regard for their personal feelings or capacity. One eminent obstetrician has recently pointed out that frustration can equal fear as a cause of tension!

However, there may be occasions when sleep-producing medications help women who have been deprived of sleep in the first stage. If dilatation is slow, two or three hours of complete rest will refresh them and they will be far better able to cope with the latter part of labour.

If contractions become very strong, analgesia can make relaxation easier. View the subject philosophically. Discuss it with your doctor or midwife. Be honest with them and with yourself, and see how you feel when the time comes. They will guide you and will know what will be the best for your individual needs.

Analgesics which are Inhaled.—It will be helpful for you to understand how efficient breathing makes this type of analgesic more effective. Nitrous-oxide gas/oxygen, and trilene, in common use to-day, are breathed into the lungs through the mouth. They pass through the walls of the lungs into tiny little blood-vessels and are carried by the blood up through the heart to the brain. On reaching the brain centres, the perceptive senses are dulled but the recipient remains fully conscious and co-operative.

It takes rather less than half a minute for these gases to make the journey from the mask, which the patient holds at will over her own face, to the brain. So you can expect to take about three to five good deep breaths of analgesic before you are aware of any relief.

The mask has a soft balloon-like edge which will fit comfortably over the nose and under the chin, whether the face is plump or thin. It should be held in firm contact all the way round. If you are lying on your side with your arm supported on the pillow, you can inhale the analgesic deeply through the mouth, and relax with a sigh or soft blow as before, thus benefiting from both aids simultaneously. It takes nearly twice as long to fill and empty the lungs through the nose as through the mouth, and therefore twice as long to get the effect.

Imagine you have run to catch a bus, and now that you have caught it you are *slightly* puffed, and breathing through your mouth. Let all the chest and shoulder muscles go slack as you breathe out and continue like this until the peak is passed. The analgesic effect will have worn off before the next contraction begins and you will be back where you started.

Points to Remember when Inhaling Analgesics.—

1. Start inhaling at the very beginning of the contraction (by now you will be familiar with the slight tightening feeling in the abdomen which heralds another wave coming), so that you have time to get the full effect before you get to the crest of the contraction. Your midwife may advise you to start even a little before a contraction is due.

54

2. Breathe easily through the mouth and continue to relax on breathing out with a sigh or soft blow.
3. Hold the mask in good contact with the face. *N.B.*: Some masks have a little vent hole at the back over which the patient is told to place her index finger. With this type of mask, if the finger is not held over the hole, the patient will not get maximum relief from the analgesia.

Spiral Descent.—

At the inlet (through which the baby descends in the early first stage) the pelvis is normally slightly wider from side to side. At the outlet (through which he passes in the second stage) it is slightly wider from front to back.

Taking the easiest route, the baby rotates with a corkscrew action as he comes round the bend and descends towards the exit (*see Fig.* 1, p. 16).

The Transition from First to Second Stage.—

The rectum, which lies immediately behind the cervix, will sooner or later be compressed by the baby's head like a piece of soft rubber tubing. This pressure makes it feel to the patient as if she wants to pass a motion, exactly the same feeling she has had many times before in her life, with a full bowel. Sometimes this desire to bear down is present before the cervix is quite fully dilated and we must continue to wait patiently, as the skipper of a large boat waits for the lock gates to open before he tries to manœuvre his boat through the lock.

It may be a good thing to sit up on the haunches, well supported with pillows, with knees bent, thighs apart, and feet flat on the bed.

Some women find that it is helpful to lift the uterus gently by stroking upward and outward from the pubic area with the palms of the hands— midwives report that women in the East often do this—and if the baby's body is tending, with the uterus, to flop forward into the abdominal muscles, his head is steered in the right direction by this type of massage. But you might prefer to remain on your side.

It is wise to delay straining down at this point, even though the desire is strong, by sighing and blowing alternately during contractions, while the uterus eases the gates open and the baby's head slides gently through the cervix.

Remember that analgesics dull all sensations, whether unpleasant or not. You may at this time be feeling no more discomfort than you would have from a full bowel, yet the analgesic can be invaluable in that it takes away some of the desire to strain down. You may in such circumstances be advised to use the mask, *not* to relieve the pain, but to reduce the inclination to exert the abdominal muscles and prevent the breath being held. This effect can be obtained by breathing through loosely parted lips, without the analgesic, and some patients prefer to manage by themselves. Others find that it is easier to keep up the rhythmical mouth-breathing if there is something positive to hold and puff and blow into. So long as the throat remains open, the chest wall and ribs are free to move and it is impossible to push.

55

There may be advantages in the sigh-blow type of breathing over the continuous pant type:—

1. It requires more concentration, which according to the Psycho-prophylactic theory is all to the good.

2. The mouth does not seem to get so dry.

3. One is less likely to do it too rapidly and shallowly,* or to over-breathe.

The Second Stage.—

Having passed through the cervix and round the bend, the baby will advance little by little with each uterine contraction, on the last part of his journey through the lower part of the birth canal. The uterus by now is very much smaller because of the shortening of the longitudinal muscle-fibres, and the contractions themselves are propelling the baby towards the world outside.

The patient feels exhilarated. She feels no stretching in the birth canal because women are built with no sensory nerves in the cervix or the upper part of the vagina. Now she knows she is getting on and she can feel the gradual advance. The pressure is felt on the rectum as if constipated, and though this can be uncomfortable, few women say that it is painful. A small minority of women do not experience the pushing urge early in the second stage. If so, the attendants will tell you when and what to do. You may find that between contractions, voices sound far away and time appears to pass much more quickly than it really does. You may feel drowsy. Give yourself up to this natural amnesia; by this resource you will be enabled to recover quickly from fatigue in labour.

Relaxation between contractions is important in the second stage. The more complete the rest during the lulls, the quicker the patient will regain strength and recover from the effects of the last effort.

As previously mentioned, the amount of power exerted by the uterus during contractions varies in individuals, so we must not have fixed ideas in our minds beforehand as to the necessity of pushing or bearing down hard in the second stage. The midwife or doctor will judge the strength of the uterus from the advance of the baby—which they will be able to see—and the patient will be instructed accordingly.

Position of Patient.—Most patients are more comfortable and better able to co-operate if they are on their backs, well propped up with a

---

* Some teachers when discussing the end of the first stage advise very shallow and rapid breathing during contractions. Others talk of panting 'like a dog'. The author has deliberately avoided these terms because she believes that adequate (but not excessive) ventilation is important for both mother and baby at that time.

Maternal Respiration in Labour, by Dr. R. St. J. Buxton, M.B., Ph.D., D.C.H., Medical Pre-clinical Dean, University of Bristol, 1969, written for the Obstetric Association of Chartered Physiotherapists. This paper gives the results of research from 1966 to 1968. The aim was to record the patterns of breathing in labour. *Extract*: 'Apical or shallow breathing is inefficient and often merely ventilates the bronchial airways. Since it does not provide adequate gas exchange in the alveoli, breathing on a shallow plane should not be allowed to persist for long periods.'

wedge-shaped back-rest or pillows under the head and shoulders as in *Fig.* 18, and in this position, breathing may be much easier, and gravity can assist the birth (half-lying). During contractions the knees and hips are bent, with thighs apart, grasped underneath, just above knees, and feet are off the bed (modified squatting). If you feel you want more pillows, ask if you may have them.

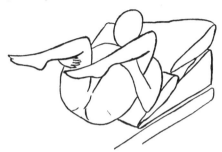

Fig. 18.—Modified squatting position for second-stage contractions.

But on this question of position, too, we should be guided by the doctor or midwife. We are individuals and so are our babies. It may be found that the progress is smoother, or that a woman benefits more from being on her side.

Breathing Control in the Second Stage.—You may be instructed during contractions, either:—

1. To take a deep breath and 'bear down' or 'push' or 'block'. The effect of this is to boost the power of expulsion:—

   a. Lungs are filled with air and the 'trap' in the throat closed.

   b. Abdominal and chest muscles are braced so that they become firm walls of the baby's 'container'.

   c. The diaphragm (supported by the ribs and the bolster of air in the lungs) pushes down in the centre (rather like a plumber's plunger) against the fundus of the uterus—which is already behaving like a forcing bag—and

   d. The baby is driven downwards and forwards through the pelvis. The more the uterus is compressed down by straining, the more the mother adds to the force of ejection.

Common Mistakes.—Some women hold their breath so long that they go blue in the face! This is not good for mother or baby. When eventually they let go, they are out of breath, and they cannot avoid gasping in another breath and drawing in the lower abdominal muscles. When this happens, the baby is drawn back up the vagina by the recoil of the 'plunger' and by the time the mother regains her respiratory control, the contraction has passed. Other women make a guttural noise while they are supposed to be holding the breath steadily. (They do not close the throat properly but make it vibrate.) This makes the throat sore and wastes effort; they should make no noise, except on letting the breath go and breathing in again.

If you are asked to 'bear down' or 'push', begin to breathe in and out deeply as soon as the contraction starts while you draw your knees up, let them fall apart, grasp behind thighs and take another deep breath expanding the ribs fully. Close the throat ('block') and with neck flexed and chin down on chest hold the air down steadily and quietly for a reasonable length of time, with pelvic floor muscles relaxed, until you feel you want to let go. Let the air go completely with neck slack, head back on pillow, and try to hold the baby down against the front of the pelvic outlet while you take another breath and repeat.

Caution.—Do not push towards the back passage. The baby (let me repeat) is coming downwards and *forwards*. Help him down that way.

Contractions may last from about $\frac{3}{4}$ to $1\frac{1}{4}$ min., and so most of us need about three breaths in these circumstances during one contraction. At the end rest the legs down, take two easy breaths and relax.

Maximum effort may or may not be required. There is no advantage in straining with the abdominal muscles if the baby is already advancing well without this exertion.

Or, if the baby is coming too quickly,

2. To breathe in and out through the mouth, lightly. This prevents voluntary expulsive effort. It may tend automatically to get quicker towards the peak of a contraction as the oxygen demand goes up and as before the pelvic floor should be relaxed.

Widening of the Pelvic Outlet.—The tail-end of the mother's spine (the coccyx) is pushed back easily by pressure on the inside, and this widens the outlet of the pelvis as the baby passes by. It springs back into its original position when the pressure has gone.

Moulding.—The baby's head is designed to enable it to narrow in diameter as it passes through the lower part of the pelvis. The little saucer-like bones of his head overlap slightly with a telescopic action (moulding), and so by a process of give and take between mother and baby the birth is accomplished more easily.

You are likely to feel hot and sticky from the effort involved, whether you are holding the breath or not. Sweetened fruit drinks are usually placed beside the bed and sipped after contractions. Your face and hands will be sponged from time to time to cool and freshen you.

Numbing.—When the baby's head reaches the pelvic floor, the urge to push usually becomes very strong. For a few moments you may be aware of the muscle stretching, but at about this point, the tissues in the surrounding locality become insensitive and remain so for about 15 min. after the birth of the baby. You remember that nerves transmit sensations to the brain? Nerves cannot work without an adequate blood-supply, and if the circulation to a sensory nerve is substantially diminished for more than a few minutes, the area supplied by that nerve becomes numb. Feet can go to sleep while their owners are wide awake, caused by pressure (probably behind the knees) and by diminished blood-supply. Hands can go numb with cold in the winter, due to constriction of blood-vessels in icy conditions. If, in such a state, you come into a warm house and the blood starts to circulate more freely, you may find that, for a short time, your hands feel burning and tingling, although they are still cold.

This same sensation is experienced when the tissues at the outlet are at the in-between stage between normal sensitivity and numbness. The advancing head will have been reducing the blood-supply and so this feeling of burning or tingling should be expected before 'crowning' of the head, and it may last for about half a minute.

The unprepared woman sometimes remarks at this point, "It feels as if I am going to split", and she may tighten up the pelvic floor muscles in resistance. An informed woman who has practised regularly will relax her pelvic floor completely and though she may choose to use the analgesic for a few moments, she is fully aware of the sequence of events. For her it is the signal that the objective for which she has been striving will probably be accomplished in a few more uterine contractions. She is ready to co-operate and follow her attendant's instruction while she *gives* birth—G-I-V-E-S !

Mothers with long legs are sometimes more comfortable with the *outsides* of the feet on the bed, by this time. If it is suggested that you might prefer to keep your feet down, make sure that the soles of the feet are not against the bed or in contact with anybody or you may get a reflex urge to push away with the feet—which is wrong.

Alternatively, you might be turned on to your left side.

Crowning.—The pelvic floor muscles have been drawn up and the widest part of the baby's head is just about to emerge. In a few moments it will be born. The doctor or midwife will want this to happen slowly and smoothly, so that there is less strain on the soft tissues. When the head is delivered, there will be a little lull when the baby rotates again—quite automatically—and the shoulders line up in the front-to-back diameter of the outlet.

Episiotomy.—It may be necessary to make a small cut in the front part of the perineum (the area between the vagina and the anus) in order to protect the pelvic floor from overstretching, prevent the possibility of a more serious tear, or ease the way for the baby. There is no inference of failure to relax or co-operate on the part of the patient, who is usually quite unaware that it is being done. She may be surprised when the birth is completed to learn that a stitch or two are necessary.

The patient cannot feel how quickly or slowly the baby is advancing and so she follows her attendant's instructions, which may be either:—

1. To take a breath and hold it steadily until crowning. Then on "That's enough", or "Stop pushing", or "Pant in and out", from her attendant, she breathes in and out softly and easily with mouth and throat open, diaphragm mobile, and ribs free while the baby's head is born, or:

2. To pant in and out from the beginning of the contraction—in the same manner, perhaps, into the mask—and keep it up until the head is born. (This would be in the case of a stronger uterine

contraction and with the aim of preventing the baby from coming too quickly.)

The Delivery.—Most women find that these last few moments are agreeably pleasant. After the shoulders have rotated, there is likely to be a repetition of one or the other of these instructions, and on the next contraction, the baby slithers gently out into the world. An injection is often given at about this time to assist the action of the uterus in the forthcoming third stage.

FIRST STAGE		
Follow natural breathing pattern, but adapt depth and rhythm to type of contr...		
When contractions become established	*When.* If contractions are strong enough to make one feel the need to breathe more quickly towards the crest	*When.* If towards of the first stage, crest of contractio... level breathing f... natural or uncom...
Position. Either:— Standing or Sitting or Half-lying or Side-lying whichever proves most comfortable	*Position.* Either:— Sitting or Half-lying or Side-lying	*Position.* Either:— Sitting or Half-lying or Side-lying
Easy Regular Low-level Breathing *How.* In calmly through nose; take air right down to bases of lungs just above waist and expand abdominal wall and lower ribs gently. Out with a sigh through nose or mouth. Link with relaxation	*Slightly Accelerated Middle-level Breathing* *How.* Lips relaxed and slightly parted. In through nose (unless there is a feeling of restriction, in which case, through mouth) expanding the middle ribs sideways—easily but a little more quickly—and Out with a sigh or soft blow through mouth. Link with relaxation	*Smooth, Rhythmica...* *level Breathing* *How.* Lips rela... In through m... panding the uppe... the rib cage (as if... run a short dis... catch a bus), and... Out with a sig... blow through mo... Do it almost eff... Link with relax... Analgesics can b... at the same time

The Third Stage.—

This is entirely the responsibility of the doctor or midwife, and the mother rests contentedly and waits for the separation of the placenta. The cord is tied and divided about three inches from the baby's abdomen, and after this, in normal deliveries, the baby is usually wrapped up and given to his mother to hold.

Many women find themselves quivering for a short time after the birth of the baby. It is the body's natural reaction to unaccustomed effort and loss of heat.

The third stage is completed with the delivery of the placenta, membranes, and the rest of the cord. Stitches, if necessary, are inserted, and if the numbness has gone and the tissues are sensitive again, care is taken to ensure that by local anæsthesia or analgesic inhalation discomfort is not felt by the patient.

A refreshing drink and a wash will be most welcome, and the mother and father will want to be alone with their new baby as soon as possible.

TRANSITION	SECOND STAGE	
f there is a desire down before the s fully dilated	*When.* During contractions, to make bearing down more effective yet less tiring. On midwife/doctor's instruction	*When* contractions are very strong or if the baby is advancing rather too quickly, to prevent voluntary expulsion, particularly during delivery of the baby's head and body. On midwife/doctor's instruction
Either:— up on haunches ing (well-suppor-pillows); or Side-	*Position.* Either:— Lying—well propped up with wedge or pillows, knees and hips bent, thighs falling apart and supported by hands underneath, just above knees; or Side-lying	*Position.* Either:— Side-lying with upper knee bent, thigh lifted; or Half-lying with knees drawn up (Both modified squatting positions)
o Mouth Breathing eathe in—sigh and ow............; h............; ow............ ut the contrac-mping neck and forward with each nphasize the out-ths slightly and let . Do it rhythmic-link with relaxa-lgesics can be in-he same time	*Bearing Down with Respiratory Blocking* *How.* As soon as contraction starts, breathe in - out, in - out fully; then breathe in again, close throat (block) and hold the compressed air down against the diaphragm steadily, until there is a strong desire to let go. Open the throat and allow the air to rush out through the mouth and immediately repeat full inspiration and 'blocking' until contraction ends. Take 2 full easy breaths	*Light Panting* *How.* Breathe in and out through the mouth like a large droopy dog on a hot day. This keeps the throat unblocked so that the diaphragm is unable to get any leverage or intensify the downward thrust of the uterus

A Summing-up.—

There seems to be little doubt among those who have experienced it that in conscious birth there is some fundamental gratification, quite apart from the pride and joy in having produced a child.

However, the natural forces of labour, the size and shape of the baby and its position in relation to the pelvis, are factors which vary in different women and even in the same woman giving birth on different occasions.

Anæsthetics and surgery are used if it becomes apparent that help is necessary. It is comforting to know that to-day competent medical aid is available to all mothers should the need arise, but that childbirth is usually natural, *even without training*, and has been for thousands of years.

After following a course of preparation no woman should judge herself, or anybody else, to be successful or not, according to the amount of attendant help that is needed in labour.

Even if assistance should be found necessary, she should bear in mind that her child has been carried under the best conditions and the aid may be less than might be required under less favourable circumstances.

V. THE RESTORATION TO FULL ACTIVITY AND WELL-BEING

It is natural to follow any big effort with complete rest. However, before you do so, you may be wise to ensure a quick return by performing two familiar exercises immediately after you have been made comfortable.

Your body needs oxygen.

Before you Settle Down to Rest.—

Make the most of your vital capacity by taking plenty of fresh air down to the bases of the lungs. Simultaneously, shorten the belt-like muscle which goes right across the abdomen from side to side and squeeze out all the stale air from the bases of the lungs, like bellows.

Exercise 1. *Low-level Breathing Plus Abdominal Retraction.*—

Positions: Lying with pillows under head and shoulders or half-lying (leaning against back-rest).

Hands placed on abdomen at waist level and knees bent up with feet flat on bed.

Movements:

1. Breathe out through the mouth while drawing the 'tummy' inwards. Go on exhaling until you can no longer make any noise with your breath and make yourself as thin as possible from front to back.
2. Breathe in through the nose, gently blowing up under your hands so that they are lifted towards the ceiling. Repeat 6 times.

Inevitably the circulation of blood in the legs and feet becomes more sluggish while labour is in progress. In our grandmother's day, movement was prohibited for some time following birth; nothing was done to quicken up the flow, and this sometimes led to circulatory complications.

To-day, early movement of toes and ankles is encouraged and so such complications have been substantially reduced.

Exercise 2. *For the Circulation.*—

Position: Lying or half-lying.

Movements: Bend and stretch the ankles about 6 times and follow by circling the feet from the ankles, 'gathering up imaginary sand' a few times.

Then relax completely and have a good rest.

Notes on the Puerperium.—

This is the period from delivery until shrinkage of the uterus is completed. Contractions of the uterus will take place from time to time for a few days, causing blood and debris to be expelled as the uterus returns to its former size and position. These contractions are usually not noticeable after a first baby but they may be more obvious after a second or subsequent child, particularly when breast-feeding. The suckling action stimulates the uterus to contract and assists its shrinkage.

When you are allowed to get out of bed for the first time, do this first: Sit with your legs hanging over the edge of the bed and before putting the feet to the ground, swing them alternately up and down from the knees a few times. This should prevent that feeling of 'pins and needles' in the feet. Then draw up the pelvic floor and hold it in contraction while you stand up and put your weight on your feet. Too-sudden changing from the horizontal to the vertical position can cause unpleasant sensations of dropping inside.

When the milk comes into the breasts ensure that they are adequately and comfortably supported.

When you sit out of bed for the first time, sit right back in the chair, with the buttocks touching the back of it and with thighs and spine supported, a cushion behind the pelvis and waist, if it is a deep arm-chair. Then relax.

Before walking for the first time, correct your standing position and try to see yourself in a mirror (*see Fig.* 3, p. 19). Walk forward with a swing from the hips and keep the pelvis balanced by maintaining some tension in the front abdominal muscles and buttocks.

When you have had a night's sleep, you will begin to think about regaining your firm muscles and adjusting yourself, now that your shape and weight distribution have changed again, to tackle your new phase of family living with comfort, poise, and enjoyment.

Two groups of muscles are stretched and weakened by carrying and bearing a child, the pelvic floor and abdominal muscles, and both should be restored to reasonable tone before a woman takes on her full everyday routine involving lifting.

If stitches have been inserted in the perineum it is advisable until they are removed to try and keep the thighs as close as possible. In the following scheme the thighs are *not* separated and therefore the exercises are usually approved medically, whether there are stitches or not.

Caution.—Strong abdominal exercises which cause a forward and downward thrust of the abdominal and pelvic organs against the weakened walls should be avoided for a few weeks, e.g., lying, lifting both legs, or trunk raising.

All the exercises suggested for your welfare before 6 weeks have an uplifting or indrawing effect, without straining.

Daytime Rest.—

Every Day.—After performing your exercises, stretch your arms, legs, and spine to the limit and then rest, face downwards, with two pillows under the pelvis and relax completely (*Fig.* 19). The position will help the abdominal and pelvic organs to fall naturally into their correct places—they are suspended from the spine—and it will feel especially comfortable to give the seat a rest for a while and allow the body-weight to be placed on some other part of the anatomy.

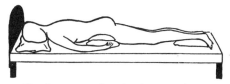

Fig. 19.—Daytime rest: relaxation in prone lying position.

On the Day following Birth (preferably during the morning, after emptying the bladder, and again in the evening).—

Repeat Exercises 1 and 2.

If you are not yet allowed to get out of bed:—

Add **Exercise 3.** *For the Quadriceps (Thigh) Muscles.* Press both knees down hard on to the bed and relax. Repeat about 6 times. (Not necessary for those who get up and use the legs in walking.)

Add **Exercise 4.** *For the Pelvic Floor Muscles.*

N.B.—Change the timing of pelvic floor movements post-natally. The accent should now be on the gradual *contraction* of the muscles. Hold for two seconds, then relax.

Sometimes the perineal area is a little congested. In this case the effect of doing the movements will be similar to squeezing and relaxing a soapy sponge in the bathwater. As one contracts, stale blood is squeezed out and as one relaxes, fresh blood flows in, cleansing and healing the tissues.

Do not worry, if you have stitches, that it might put a strain on them. In fact it will draw the edges closer together.

Sometimes the mechanism of control through interaction between nerve and muscle in the pelvic area is slightly confused for a day or two. It is not uncommon, at first, to have a little difficulty with passing water and 'retracting the undercarriage'. If this is the case, the mere attempting of Pelvic Floor contractions will hasten your return to normal. *The exercise should be repeated at frequent intervals throughout the day.*

Position: Lying down or half-sitting up in bed with knees bent and thighs slightly apart, feet flat on bed. It can be done while reading, knitting, serving, or at odd moments when you are doing nothing special.

Movements:

1. Lift, squeeze, and draw the back passage upward as if to draw air inside. Relax and repeat 3 times.
2. Squeeze the front passage forward against the pubic bone, as if to control the bladder. Relax and repeat 3 times.

3. Try to draw the vagina up inside towards the abdomen. Relax and repeat 3 times.

When you are allowed to get up, you can do it in sitting and, later on, in standing when actively engaged in cooking, preparing the vegetables, arranging the flowers, dusting, or talking on the telephone. Make it a habit, always to draw up the pelvic floor after emptying the bladder or the rectum, coughing, sneezing, or bearing down in any way.

Second and Third Day after Birth.—
Repeat Exercises 1 and 4. (Exercises 2 and 3 should be kept up if you have poor circulation or have to remain in bed.)

Add **Exercise 5.**—Pelvic Uptilting (for the centre front of 'tummy ').
Position: Lying on the back, both knees bent and slightly apart, feet flat on bed.

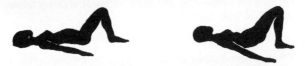

Fig. 20.—Pelvic uptilting: lying with knees bent.

Movements:
1. Press the waist down on the bed and tilt the pelvis up in front towards the ribs. Hold for a second.
2. Relax and allow the spine to hollow at the waist, naturally.
   Repeat 6 times. (*Fig.* 20.)

Add **Exercise 6.**—Hip Shrugging (for the sides of the waist).

Position: Lying on the back with one knee bent and one straight.

Movements:
1. Draw the hip of the straight leg up towards the ribs on the same side (leg seems shorter).

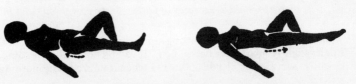

Fig. 21.—Hip shrugging, lying on back, one knee bent.

2. Stretch it out again to the utmost (leg seems longer).
   Repeat 6 times with each leg. (*Fig.* 21.)

Add **Exercise 7.**—Pelvic Rotation (for the criss-cross muscles).

66

Position: Lying on back, both knees bent and together, feet flat on bed and arms out sideways, hands holding the edges of the mattress.

Movements:

1. Swing both knees to the left and twist pelvis until the right hip is uppermost.
2. Swing to the right and twist pelvis until the left hip is uppermost.
   Keep knees together and shoulders flat on bed all the time. Do not stop. Keep swinging alternate ways.
   Repeat 6 times in each direction. (*Fig. 22.*)

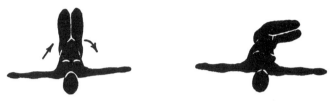

Fig. 22.—Pelvic rotation. Lying on back, knees bent, feet on floor.

Rhythm.—

Perform each of these movements smoothly and thoroughly so that the stretched muscles are contracted to their limit each time. If the timing is too quick, it is impossible to finish the movements and the muscle-fibres are not fully shortened. In the early days it is better to be slow, making the maximum effort and then trying to go a little bit farther. As tone and strength return, it will become easier to combine speed with full contraction.

Graduate the exercises, until full strength is regained, by increasing the load on your muscles. Make progressions on the basic abdominal and pelvic movements by changing the starting positions and by gradually increasing the number of repetitions by one per day to a maximum of 20.

Always stop short if you are feeling tired.

Fourth Day after Birth.—

As for third day but now seven repetitions for Exercises 5, 6, and 7.

Fifth Day after Birth.—

Perform Exercises 1 and 4 as before, but change your starting position for Exercises 5 and 6:—

Exercise 5.—Pelvic Uptilting (Progression). (*Fig. 23.*)

Fig. 23.—Pelvic uptilting: prone kneeling.

Position: Prone kneeling on bed.

Movements:

1. Tilt the pelvis up in front towards the ribs and press the waist up towards the ceiling (round back, seat tucked down and under). Hold for a second.
2. Relax and allow the spine to hollow naturally. Repeat 8 times. Rest for half a minute on forearms and knees.

Exercise 6.—Hip Shrugging (Progression).

Position: Prone kneeling, one leg stretched out straight behind, toes touching floor.

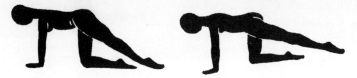

Fig. 24.—Hip shrugging, prone kneeling, one leg extended.

Movements:

1. Draw the hip of the straight leg up towards the ribs on the same side and make it as short as possible by tilting the pelvis sideways.
2. Stretch it out again (long leg). Repeat 8 times with each leg. Rest down on forearms and knees for half a minute. (*Fig.* 24.)

Exercise 7.—Pelvic Rotation. Continue as before (8 times).

Add **Exercise 8**: For the Pectoral Muscles.—*See* p. 45.

If breast-feeding, do both movements after feeds when the breasts are lighter. *N.B.* : If they are very congested, omit this exercise until comfortable.

Sixth to Seventeenth Day after Birth.—

As for the fifth day, increasing repetitions for Exercises 5, 6, and 7 from 9 to 20 times (maximum) by one daily.

Correct your posture while standing and sitting, now and again, each day. Look in a mirror to do this if you can.

Encourage your uterus to return to its correct position. Your midwife will have been checking its involution (shrinkage) and when it can no longer be felt above the brim of the pelvis in front, it can more easily be tipped into its correct forward-tilted position, because it is less bulky. The position of prone kneeling with forearms on bed or floor is particularly effective both for doing this and for uplifting the pelvic and abdominal organs (*see Fig.* 8, p. 26).

Still continue to rest in the prone lying position every day after your exercises, at least until you have had your post-natal check-up at six weeks after delivery.

Eighteenth to Thirtieth Day after Birth.—

Exercise 1. Modify it. Pull your 'tummy' in and hold it on six different occasions during the day, while you continue breathing in and out naturally, talking or even singing to yourself. Do it while talking on the telephone, if you have one.

Exercise 4. Continue as before with pelvic floor contractions.

Exercise 5.—Pelvic Uptilting (further progression).

Position: Lying on back on a rug, both knees bent and slightly apart feet flat on floor.

Movements:
1. Press the waist on floor and tilt the pelvis up in front.
2. *Holding the pelvis up-tilted,* curl the trunk and lift the shoulders upward and forward (bringing the ribs nearer to the front of the

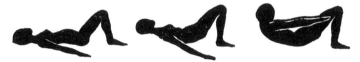

Fig. 25.—Pelvic uptilting plus lifting head and shoulders, trying to touch knees with finger-tips.

pelvis) while keeping the waist on the floor. Try to touch the knees with the finger-tips.
3. Hold for a second or two.
4. Relax and return to starting position.
   Repeat 10 times, rest for half a minute, then repeat another 10 times (20 in all). (*Fig.* 25.)

Exercise 6.—Hip Shrugging (further progression).

Position: Sitting upright with legs straight (long sitting) and arms away from body to the sides, finger-tips or palms resting on floor.

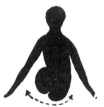

Fig. 26.—Long sitting : buttock rolling.

Movements: Tilt the pelvis up on alternate sides, lifting as high as possible, towards the ribs and rolling on the buttocks.

Repeat to each side 10 times. Rest for half a minute, then repeat another 10 times (20 in all). (*Fig.* 26.)

Exercise 7.—Pelvic Rotation (progression). Continue as before but with a cushion between knees.

Exercise 8.—Continue the pectoral exercise after breast-feeding or, if the baby is not breast-fed, at any convenient time of day.

One Month to Six Weeks after Birth.—

Exercise 1, continue as a postural exercise. (As on p. 69.)

Exercise 4, continue as before. Pelvic floor contractions should be becoming a habit by now.

Add the 'Bath' Exercise.—

Position: When taking a bath, lie in the water with legs bent, thighs rotated outwards and resting against the sides of the bath. Place a finger inside the vagina about $1\frac{1}{2}$ inches.

Movements:

1. Contract the pelvic floor as if trying to stop passing water. Feel the grip of the inside edges of the muscles against the finger and endeavour to draw it up inside.
2. Let it go.
   Repeat 6 times. The finger gives resistance and a tactile aid. Muscles work better against resistance and each time the exercise is performed you will be enabled to assess the slight improvement in power.

Exercises 5, 6, and 7. Perform the movements as for eighteenth to thirtieth day after birth but progress to three repetitions of 10, with a half-minute rest in between each (30 in all).

Corsets v. Girdles.—Do not allow yourself to be persuaded that because you have had a baby you need boned corsets. This view is quite outmoded. In fact if you *do* wear bones to do the supporting for which Nature provided you with muscles, she will probably get her own back! Any part of the body which is not used will deteriorate and waste. The muscles will let go and rely on the corset to do their job for them. The figure may look reasonably good when the corset is on, but not when it is removed. Muscles, unlike corsets, improve with constant use.

However, until full muscle tone is restored, you are advised to wear a resilient girdle of two-way stretch elastic or 'Lycra', of either the straight or the criss-cross type, for comfort. It will give some support, but your muscles will still have to work inside. When outline and strength are back to pre-pregnancy standards (or better) this girdle can be replaced by a suspender belt or discarded, if you prefer to go without, but always wear a brassière when up and about.

Comfort and Support when Breast-feeding.—The baby should rest snugly on his mother's lap to feed and the mother should be able to relax, fully supported with her back straight while she is nursing.

Sometimes, if the breasts are placed high on the chest, it is better for mother and child if a pillow is placed on the lap to lift the baby nearer to the nipple. Baby should never be allowed to drag downwards on the breasts and the mother should not round her shoulders in an effort to bring the nipple down to the baby's level.

Prams and Pram-pushing.—Choose the pram carefully. The height of the handle in relation to the pusher is one of the important considerations. You should be able to push without bending forward. Adjustable handles are ideal, but wrist-level or just above is usually comfortable.

If it is necessary at any time to draw a pram up steps, remember to bend the knees, and keep the spine straight with the head back. Use the body-weight and the thigh muscles to do the lifting. A patient who recently needed treatment for a slipped disk had suddenly suffered intense pain when dragging her pram up steps with straight legs and bent back.

Back to Routine Duties.—

On return home from hospital or nursing home, or when the midwife leaves, most mothers feel happy and contented, but there is likely to be a more pronounced awareness of responsibility.

During pregnancy and for a short while after birth, the hormone balance of the body is unsettled and this can have an unsettling effect on our emotional stability. After all the congratulations and fuss of the first week or so, there may be a feeling of anti-climax. Do not worry, nor let your husband do so, if you feel depressed on occasions for no real reason. This is not unusual and it has probably happened to most of your friends and relations, even if they have not mentioned it to you. Both the ups and downs seem to be accentuated at this time but the moods settle down to a smoother rhythm very shortly.

Looking after a baby single-handed takes a lot more time and energy at first than it does later on when parents are more adept and familiar with the sort of noises a baby makes when he is hungry, uncomfortable, or just wanting attention.

When you take on the responsibility of running the home once more, plan your day to be as simple as possible. For the time being, do only the jobs which are essential, so that you have more time to share with your husband and vigour to have fun with the baby, as well as to look after his needs and comforts.

Try to arrange to have your own rest and leisure and to follow your personal interests and recreations when the baby is asleep.

You may find it more beneficial and convenient, from now on, to do your exercises after the baby's afternoon feed and then relax for an hour on the bed.

Follow the suggestions in the section on POSTURE, POISE, AND COMFORT IN DAILY LIVING (p. 19) and, once you have developed the habit of managing your body with ease and grace, keep it for the rest of your life.

Medical Check-up.—It is advisable for all women to have a post-natal examination approximately 6 weeks after giving birth. This includes an assessment of the tone of the abdominal and pelvic floor muscles. Make a point of asking about this.

If the tone is good and everything is in order then you can, with safety, resume all activities to the full. You will not need to continue with organized exercises beyond this point.

But if your doctor considers that your tone is insufficient you should continue.

Our mothers and grandmothers often suffered unnecessary discomfort and embarrassment for years because they had a minor prolapse—due simply to weakness of the pelvic floor muscles.

After the check-up, a few women still complain of feeling 'weighed down' or 'achey' underneath the pelvis; others complain of lack of sexual appreciation or even that intercourse hurts!

The sensory nerve-endings which are so important to us women in sexual participation are situated within the pelvic floor (you will recall that there are no such nerves—and therefore no feeling—in the cervix or the upper part of the vagina) so sometimes these muscles just cannot respond as they might. They should be relaxed and willingly receptive, but before the climax they should be able to give little embracing contractions.

A slack, unresponsive pelvic floor is often the cause of dissatisfaction for *both* partners, but an understanding of their function can lead to better tone with increased perception and contentment.

Many young mothers have found themselves unable to control their bladder on stress (i.e., when sneezing, coughing, or running). With good effect they might try again and again that game that most of us remember playing as small children while passing water: stop—go—stop—go.

In all the situations mentioned, women can, by their own efforts, regain complete control and self-confidence by continuing to improve the power in their pelvic supportive muscles.

So, if any of them apply to you, don't worry! Just keep on doing your homework.

Your Figure.—

You might be told by your doctor that everything is all right but your figure may still not come up to your own standards. Very few of us, by 6 weeks after a birth, can get into our pre-maternity clothes—which fitted us a year before—and feel comfortable.

In that case, drop all the previous exercises and have a complete change for that last bit of toning up and fining down. (If you are still breast-feeding, wait until you wean the baby.)

Extra layers of fat deposited around the hips, waist, and thighs during pregnancy should gradually be absorbed, providing you watch and limit your intake of starches and sugars (chocolates, cakes, bread, cereals, pastry, chips, etc.). The fatty tissue will break down more readily with a renewed attack—daily doses of the following movements:—

To Trim the Thighs.—

Position: Forward lying on the rug with face on hands, knees bent to a right angle.

Movement: Lift one thigh at a time high up and bump down rhythmically on the floor.

Repeat until the hams start to ache. Stop. (*Fig. 27.*)

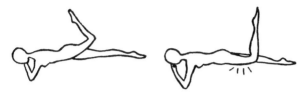

Fig. 27.

To Firm the Flanks and Pare the Hips.—

Position: Lying on back on the rug, knees bent, feet flat on floor.

Movements: Lift pelvis off the floor, then twist it and lower to bump alternative sides of your seat on the floor. (*Fig. 28.*)

1. Lift pelvis—twist—bump left buttock.
2. Lift pelvis—twist—bump right buttock.

This is self-massage! Much more effective than the expensive mechanical vibrators and shakers.

Fig. 28.

To Eliminate a ' Kangaroo Pouch' Below the Navel and a ' Tyre' Above it.—

Position: Lying on back on the rug or carpet, legs up with ankles wrapped around the arm of a chair (padded), heels resting on top.

Movement: Keeping the waist pressed down on the floor, hold tightly with the ankles, press the thighs together, and lift your head and shoulders up, reaching forward with finger-tips towards knees. Hold for a second or two, then lower. Repeat until it begins to ache in front of your waist. Stop. (*Fig. 29.*)

(You will feel that you are lifting the pelvic floor and working your front abdominal muscles at the same time.)

73

To Whittle the Waist.—

Position: Standing with your right side towards a wall, feet apart, back straight.

Movements: Bring left arm up and over the top of the head, fingers reaching towards the wall. Right arm moves *down* at the side, fingers reaching towards knee.

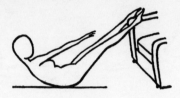

Fig. 29.

It is important to move sideways and not to turn at all. You should feel the strong contractions of the waist muscles on the right and stretching on the left side.

Give little rhythmical thrusts, starting about 6 times, then turn to face the other way—reach down on left side—up and over to the wall stretching right side. Increase gradually. (*Fig.* 30.)

If you can touch the wall easily, move farther away.

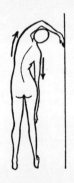

Fig. 30.

The measure of your success will be in the ultimate result at the end of the childbearing cycle. When breast-feeding has terminated and the body has settled down to its usual rhythm, you can be AT YOUR BEST and look it.